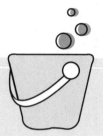

CLEAN MAMA'S GUIDE
TO A HEALTHY HOME

CLEAN MAMA'S GUIDE TO A HEALTHY HOME

The Simple, Room-by-Room
Plan for a Natural Home

BECKY RAPINCHUK

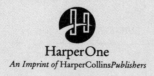

HarperOne
An Imprint of HarperCollinsPublishers

HarperOne

HarperCollins books may be purchased for educational, business, or sales promotional use. For information, please email the Special Markets Department at SPsales@harpercollins.com.

FIRST EDITION

Designed by Janet Evans-Scanlon
Illustrations by Bekah Williamson

Library of Congress Cataloging-in-Publication Data
Names: Rapinchuk, Becky, author.
Title: Clean mama's guide to a healthy home : the simple, room-by-room plan
   for a natural home / Becky Rapinchuk.
Description: First edition. | San Francisco : HarperOne, 2019 | Includes
   bibliographical references.
Identifiers: LCCN 2018036756 (print) | LCCN 2018038317 (ebook) | ISBN
   9780062856333 (e-book) | ISBN 9780062856319 (pbk.)
Subjects: LCSH: Home economics. | House cleaning. | Orderliness. |
   Do-it-yourself work.
Classification: LCC TX158 (ebook) | LCC TX158 .R36 2019 (print) | DDC
   648/.5—dc23
LC record available at https://lccn.loc.gov/2018036756

---

19 20 21 22 23   LSC   10 9 8 7 6 5 4 3 2 1

For my husband and kids. You make everything better.

Contents

An Invitation to a Better Way of Cleaning

I've always been a bit obsessive about cleaning. Years ago, I was an art teacher at an elementary school, and let me tell you, no one knows messes like art teachers. I was surrounded by dozens of sticky, splattered, paint-and-glue-covered six-year-olds each day, and it was my job to get them playing with art supplies and perfectly cleaned up in a forty-five-minute class period. I'd already had my share of kiddo-transmitted illnesses, and so I wasn't about to waste precious days off sick with the flu or a cold. So my motto became: disinfect *everything*.

I waged a war on germs, using a water-and-bleach solution, disinfecting wipes, and disinfecting spray as my daily weapons. The stronger the product, the more I trusted it to keep my students and myself clean and healthy. I can remember discussing different cleaners with my parent helpers, and we all agreed: the stronger, the better and the more germs eradicated and out of our lives. Kids even brought in disinfecting wipes as part of their supply list. I gladly added these to my stash and knew I could get rid of any germ that came my way.

Maybe this sounds familiar to you. Maybe you've been part of Team Disinfectant Spray too. Maybe you have an arsenal of sprays hidden in your hall closet. I get it. It feels good to be armed against germs. But I ended up throwing almost all my sprays away after a scary moment with my daughter.

When our first child was born, my germaphobia increased, and my "Disinfect *everything*" motto ruled our house. I blame hormones and my heightened protection instinct. It was no longer a matter of protecting just my health but also the health of my sweet baby and her developing immune system. My stash of cleaning products drastically increased, and I desperately fought to create a safe living environment, free of harmful bacteria and germs.

I was cleaning my daughter's high chair when she was about a year old and placed the bottle of all-purpose cleaner on her chair. She snatched the bottle, held it up, and sprayed it directly onto her chest, neck, and face like perfume, happily inhaling the scent. Horrified, I grabbed the spray out of her hand and wiped her clothes with a paper towel, hoping it hadn't stained her outfit. I didn't think too much about what was on her skin until I glanced at the back of the bottle. It was covered in warning signs in the tiniest font explaining how toxic the contents were. How had I not noticed this before?! This was the fancy spray that I'd paid more for because the commercials promised it was safe for kids and could be used to clean toys, high chairs, counters—everywhere kids make their biggest messes. The commercials also touted that it didn't need to be rinsed. In my mind, no need to rinse indicated that it was safe and effective.

I heeded the toxicity warnings and, in a full-blown panic, started making frantic calls to Poison Control, dunking my daughter in a warm bath, giving her milk to settle her stomach, nervously examining her for signs of a rash or allergic reaction, and spending the next twenty-four hours watching her closely, hoping she wouldn't be one of the 7 percent who dies or is severely affected by toxin exposure. (If you want to take a few years off your life, spend some time on the Poison Control website.)

Fortunately, no rash appeared, a middle-of-the-night ER visit was never necessary, and my baby girl seemed her happy and healthy self the next day. But those moments of panic stuck with me, and I couldn't shake the feeling that there was something wrong—very wrong—with what had just happened.

Starting that day, I learned more about cleaning products, and I found that the products I thought were safe and keeping my family healthy were actually toxic. This is what really makes me angry: we pay to bring harmful toxins into our homes. Think about that for a second. I'm not talking about your baby spraying something on his or her face and neck; I'm talking about the use of these products for normal, everyday cleaning. When you wash your hands with a simple hand soap to get rid of germs, you add artificial fragrance and possibly formaldehyde onto your skin. I'm not telling you this to send you into a full-on panic. We are all doing our best to take care of our families and provide safe, healthy spaces for them. I just want to help you in that task— that's why you're reading this book! I'm going to show you how to decipher ingredient labels and find or make products that are truly *safe* and *effective*.

I can't wait to share what I've learned about homekeeping through the years, including my program for making cleaning approachable and, best of all, fit into your busy life. This book will help you simplify your cleaning in the best possible way— naturally. You'll streamline your routine, declutter, and make your home safe, all at the same time.

My cleaning philosophy has been refined over my years of working multiple jobs and having three kids as well as dogs. I support safe, nontoxic cleaning products and have shared natural cleaning recipes on my blog, where I also share my struggles with keeping things clean while still enjoying my family. If you've followed me from the start, you may have noticed that I don't recommend the same products I used to, but my mission is still the same: clean with the simplest products you can until you find something better and/or safer. This book is a glimpse behind the scenes of my journey. It contains information I've distilled over years of research, testing, experimentation, and just putting things to use day in and day out in our home. A clean and nearly germ-free home can be attained without using toxic products and chemicals.

If you've followed me on my website or read my books, I'm so glad you're taking this next step with me! Hopefully you've found a cleaning routine that works well for your schedule and your family; the information in this book will supplement what you're already doing and improve the way you're cleaning.

If you're new to the community, welcome! I'm excited to take this journey with you.

I'll help you navigate this confusing, and often scary, landscape. As we delve into the research about toxins and dangerous products, I don't want you to feel nervous or afraid—I'll give you very clear instructions and action steps that you can take *today* to make your home and your family safer. I only ask that you put aside any preconceptions you have about what "clean" really is and read with an open mind. I've been on this health and wellness journey for a decade, and I can assure you that with a handful of simple changes, you too will be on your way to a healthy home.

We'll start by detoxing your home of unsafe cleaning products. I've found that the best place to begin this is with home care products. By choosing safe products, you'll get the most beneficial change right away. I'll help you take an inventory of your cleaning supplies and decide what needs to go. The best part of this detox is that you may even notice a difference in the air quality of your home *just* from removing a couple of key ingredients. If you're busy (who isn't?), the quick Kick-Start Weekend Detox is where to begin. In just one weekend, you'll clear the air in your home, make an all-purpose cleaner that you can use on just about everything, and learn how one word—"fragrance"—can change your whole home.

After you feel like you can breathe again, literally and figuratively, we'll go from room to room and discover some simple swaps you can make to replace what you may think you cannot live without. I've found that eliminating products only works if I have a replacement that works just as well or better. It's kind of like a no-sugar diet: if you're trying to give up sugar, you need some sweet things to replace the food items you count on. Spinach doesn't taste like something sweet, but add a banana or an apple to that green smoothie, and you can't taste the spinach anymore. So room by room we'll examine the different products: those that are definitely harmful, those that are not as bad, and those you can change down the road when you're ready to replace an item. Through this process, I'll teach you how to determine the safety of any product in a hurry, and I'll share my favorite alternative products and home-made recipes.

Are you ready? Together, we're going to give your home a natural detox and begin your journey toward a better way of cleaning. My simple routine paired with the right products is magic. There are countless benefits—to your family's health, the state of your home, and just your peace of mind—so let's begin!

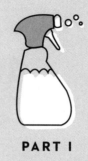

PART I

THE PROBLEM WITH CLEAN

CHAPTER 1

Is Your Home Making You Sick?

YEARS AGO, WHEN WE WERE GETTING OUR TOWN HOUSE READY TO SELL, I WAS TRYING to get rid of some soap scum in one of the bathrooms. I grabbed a soap-scum cleaner, sprayed the tub down, and walked away to let the cleaner do its thing. Minutes later, the smell from the second-floor bathroom was so strong, even with the bathroom door closed and the fan on, I had to quickly rinse off the cleaner, throw open the little bathroom window, and pile the kids into the car to go somewhere while we waited for the smell to dissipate. This was one of the moments that opened my irritated eyes, nose, and throat to what cleaners really contain. I started thinking back to other cleaners that had caused irritation: oven cleaners, cleaners with bleach, bathroom cleaners, drain cleaners. Why was it okay to use cleaners like these all the time, except when you were pregnant, when the doctor warned against it? Why was it not safe for pregnant women and children to be near these cleaners but it was okay for adults?

Looking back, I had a gut feeling at the time that these cleaners weren't the best to be using, but I countered that thought with the importance of having a disinfected bathroom or kitchen counter. The headaches and burning eyes were worth the cost so my babies had sparkling floors to crawl on and clean toilets to sit on. I thought I needed to use the strongest cleaners possible to keep my family safe. My worst nightmare was spreading the stomach flu around the house, so if a cleaner singed my nose hairs, I thought it must be really effective and could eradicate those stomach-flu germs!

Maybe, like I once did, you think that the stronger the smell, the better the cleaner. If you or someone you know has ever had a reaction to a household product, which can range from a mild headache all the way to poisoning, you know something in that cleaner, air freshener, detergent, or wall paint isn't good for your body. Our bodies are designed to react to things that aren't good for us. Eat bad shellfish, your body knows how to get rid of it. A noxious odor will cause you to pinch your nose, open a window, or leave the room. These reactions are helpful—but what if you don't smell something? Or what if you're so used to using certain products that a reaction no longer occurs? Or what if some people react differently than others? Is that product still harmful? Is it affecting someone in your home? Could the effects linger, silently making you sick? What are the regulations on chemicals? Haven't commercial products been tested to make sure they're safe for consumers to use in their homes?

Twenty Questions About Toxins

These are the questions I had that kept me up at night and made me wonder what was really in that blue bottle I used to disinfect the toilet, the questions that led me to methodically reconsider everything I was bringing into our home. When I first started taking notice of chemicals in the home, I considered only cleaning products. But did you know that thousands of chemicals currently used in products on store shelves have never been tested for safety? The Toxic Substances Control Act of 1976, regarding chemicals in household products, grandfathered in thousands of chemicals existing in the United States at the time, classifying them all as safe. The act states that new chemicals and ingredients are tested only when there is a concern over their safety. An updated act, the Lautenberg Chemical Safety Act, was passed in 2016, but all it considers are ten chemicals—not the thousands that are still untested.[1]

What does that really mean? Until people get sick, companies are not concerned about the safety of either new or existing chemicals in their household products. Food, drugs, and pesticides are more strictly regulated than household products. According to the Natural Resources Defense Council (NRDC)—a nonprofit, nonpartisan research group that has been working to make the world a little safer since the 1970s—more than 80,000 chemicals used in household products have not been thoroughly tested.[2] For me, knowing that many household chemicals haven't been tested,[3] I'm going to find out what *is* safe and what *has* been tested and start there. I won't wait for someone to test each and every one of those products, because clearly it isn't a priority.

I was overwhelmed with just these initial findings and not sure who to believe or what I should do. So I started small and did what I could to clear our home of toxic cleaners. I threw out any questionable products and started cleaning with simply dish soap and water. I figured if my grandma used that to clean just about everything, it must be an okay place to start. Counters, bathtubs, sinks—I used it on anything that needed a good scrubbing. The soap-and-water method worked really well on most surfaces and was easy to use. But then I looked at the label on the dish soap and saw there were cautions on that too. *You have got to be kidding me!* I used this on all our dishes. Was it safe to eat off our dishes? That led me to look at the dishwashing detergent I used, and you guessed it: CAUTION, CAUTION, CAUTION. Did this rinse off? Should I worry about it? Or were we eating a little bit of these toxic ingredients with every bite?

The Power of Google

I next did what any clearheaded, rational mom would do: I went down the internet rabbit hole and Googled, then Googled some more. There's a lot of information out there, and sifting through it all to find what's accurate and what the reputable sources are can be tricky. Finally I found a couple of organizations doing extensive research in order to figure out what was safe and what wasn't. I cross-referenced and found some information that made sense and quite a bit that didn't. The most helpful website was EWG.org. The Environmental Working Group tests and rates products for toxicity and potential side effects, and their website is an incredible database of knowledge and resources. I highly recommend typing your favorite cleaning product into their search engine. Assuming the product is listed, EWG grades the product, A to F, and tells you why it gives it that grade, which allows you to make an informed decision.

Another place to check out is MadeSafe.org. According to their website, Made Safe is an organization that "provides America's first comprehensive human health-focused certification for nontoxic products across store aisles, from baby to personal care to household and beyond."[4] The website lists their certified and approved products and brands, and while unfortunately the list isn't very long, you'll most likely find some new products to try.

Lastly, I recommend downloading the Think Dirty app (from ThinkDirtyApp .com). With this, you can scan or type in a product, and it rates it from 0 to 10—0 being the best, 10 the worst. It's not always perfectly accurate—I've seen good (and bad) product ratings that I disagreed with—but it's a place to start.

Environmental Working Group, Made Safe, and Think Dirty are all excellent resources for determining if a product is safe to use.

It has been more than ten years since I began this cleaning "adventure," and surprisingly, not a lot has changed when it comes to the many toxic products available, but there are a lot more options for "natural" and "green" household products. Having more choices is good for consumers, but it also makes it more confusing because there are new, unfamiliar ingredients, and new names for the same ingredients. Also, quite a few of the companies that were small and independent ten to fifteen years ago have been bought by big companies, which sell other household products that aren't safe. What does this mean? Generally, the smaller companies still produce their own products, but it's much more important for consumers to watch the ingredients. Companies change formulations all the time—sometimes to reformulate something to meet new safety guidelines, sometimes because they've found a more effective ingredient, sometimes to use cheaper ingredients, or just to introduce a new seasonal scent. Companies often changing their formulations without notice, combined with the industry standard that products don't need to be tested until after they've been found to be harmful, has never sat well with me. But I couldn't even begin to think about anything else until I had gone through my own products and "cleaned up" that part of our home.

I focused on tossing the harmful cleaners, but as I kept researching, I found that so many home care, household, beauty, and personal products have harmful ingredients and produce side effects. Frightened, I started second-guessing everything in our home, which is a terrible way to live! I don't want you to feel uninformed or that you don't have choices for a naturally clean home. My hope is that this book will help you feel empowered with knowledge so you can rest assured your home is truly clean and safe.

Should You Worry About Pollution Inside Your Home?

Home care and household products have radically changed in the past fifty years, and the average American comes into contact with hundreds of chemicals, pesticides, carcinogens, and toxins every single day at home. Recent research by the EPA shows that indoor air is two to five times more polluted or toxic than outside air, even in the most polluted cities. Since Americans spend 90 percent of their time indoors, the EPA calls the current state of indoor air quality a "serious risk."[5] Why is the air so polluted in *our own homes*?

When I hear "pollution," I think smog-filled cities and people walking around with those disposable face masks, not my living room. But a 2018 study done by researchers at the University of Bergen in Norway, which followed more than six thousand women over the course of twenty years, found a correlation between decreased lung function and the use of cleaning products over time. The findings were clear: people who clean using conventional cleaning products might face decreased lung function and damage. "The take home message of this study," Øistein Svanes—one of the researchers—said, "is that in the long run, cleaning chemicals very likely cause rather substantial damage to your lungs. These chemicals are usually unnecessary; microfiber cloths and water are more than enough for most purposes."[6]

In my opinion, there is no counter or toilet that deserves to take away my lung function.

New information comes out daily about household chemicals, pesticides, and other toxins and the effects they have on our overall health and immune system. It's no surprise that allergies and asthma rates are up and that studies are showing links between household chemicals and cancer, arthritis, lupus, chronic fatigue syndrome, multiple sclerosis, Alzheimer's, Parkinson's disease, and other chronic illnesses, and these diseases continue to be on the rise.[7] This is so upsetting but not surprising once you start looking into what's in the products we use every day.

Mothers also pass these chemicals on to their babies in utero and through breast milk. The US Department of Health and Human Services has found chemicals like lead and pesticides, as well as the chemicals found in Teflon and Scotchgard, in newborn baby umbilical cord blood. According to the EWG, "of the 287 chemicals we detected in umbilical cord blood, we know that 180 cause cancer in humans or animals, 217 are toxic to the brain and nervous system, and 208 cause birth defects or abnormal development in animal tests. The dangers of pre- or post-natal exposure to this complex mixture of carcinogens, developmental toxins, and neurotoxins have never been studied."[8]

These are scary facts. But now that you know them, you have the power to do something to avoid being part of the statistics. If the air inside our homes is two to five times more polluted than the outside air in the most polluted cities, we need to take a look at what we're bringing into our homes. That's on us. We can't necessarily control the companies that emit pollutants from their exhaust systems or let chemicals seep into the ground, but we can control what we put into our shopping carts and under our sinks.

Let's figure out a better, safe, *and* effective way to clean our homes, shall we?

Lots of Feelings

I realize the statistics are frightening and difficult to read. It can be easier to ignore them, but wouldn't you rather face the challenge now than deal with health issues later?

You may also be starting to wonder if this is really worth the effort. I know how it feels to say to yourself "Maybe next year, when I have more free time" or "I'll worry about it when the kids are older and I can concentrate for more than thirty seconds on any given thing." This is where I want to help! In the pages of this book I've done the research for you, and I offer a plan to easily put what you'll learn into practice.

You also may be feeling nervous, or even like keeping yourself and your family safe is a losing battle. While I don't want you to feel powerless or out of control, recognizing that you feel nervous can make you aware that there's a problem to address, and once you realize that, you're ready to make a change.

Instead of fear or worry or concern that it's too much effort, I suggest that you get excited! You're about to embark on a new way of living. You'll soon be able to edit the products you already have in your home with ease, knowing what's safe and what isn't. Take confidence in the fact that you'll be making safe and sound choices with every product you bring into your home!

CHAPTER 2

What Is in Your Cleaning Supplies?

WHAT DOES YOUR CLEANING STASH LOOK LIKE? IF YOU'RE LIKE MOST PEOPLE, YOU probably have an all-purpose cleaner, a toilet cleaner, a shower cleaner, and a sink scrub. You probably also have laundry detergent, dish soap, and dryer sheets. You might even have a gallon of bleach or a jug of ammonia somewhere. And now I'm going to tell you that it's important to go through all your cleaners and throw everything away. (Contact your local hazardous waste facility for proper disposal.)

Yes, everything. And you're going to think that I'm crazy, and you're going to wonder how much you can get for this book if it's not really used. I'm kidding, but realistically you probably have a doubt or two (or twelve). I'm here to tell you that I wish I'd had the confidence to just chuck everything when I started down this path all those years ago. I hope you trust that what I'm sharing with you will make your home *clean* and keep your family *healthy,* and you'll be *safer* than before you implemented anything in this book.

In chapter 6, I'll take you through a painless Kick-Start Weekend Detox, where we'll go through each of your cleaning supplies and get rid of the ones that are toxic. But before we get there, I want you to understand *why* they're so toxic. Let's start by taking a look at what's actually in the products you use every day. Spoiler alert: most conventional cleaning products have at least one harmful chemical ingredient on the list.

What's Actually *in* This Stuff?

Here's a simple list of common household cleaners and just a few of the typical ingredients you'll find in them. Each ingredient listed is rated C, D, or F by the Environmental Working Group. (Later in the chapter I'll take you through most of these ingredients to show you what they are and why they're harmful.)

LAUNDRY DETERGENT
linear alkylbenzene sulfonate, sulfates, fragrance, benzisothiazolinone, methylisothiazolinone

HAND SOAP
sulfates, fragrance, benzisothiazolinone, methylisothiazolinone, ethanolamine, FD&C Yellow 5

FABRIC SOFTENER AND DRYER SHEETS
fragrance, benzyl acetate, benzyl alcohol, ethanol, limonene

DISH SOAP
sulfates, fragrance, benzisothiazolinone, methylisothiazolinone

DISINFECTANT
ethanolamine, FD&C Yellow 5, fragrance, alkyl dimethyl benzyl ammonium

CLEANING/ DISINFECTING WIPES
fragrance, alkyl dimethyl benzyl ammonium chlorides (C12–16)

DUSTING POLISH
fragrance, butane, isobutane, propane

DISHWASHER DETERGENT
fragrance, sodium polyacrylate, tetrasodium etidronate, tolyltriazole

BLEACH
sodium hypochlorite

TOILET CLEANER
fragrance, sodium hydroxide, alcohol ethoxylates

WINDOW/MIRROR SPRAY
ammonium hydroxide, hexoxyethanol, fragrance, sodium borate

CARPET CLEANER
fragrance, acrylic acid, sodium salts, methylisothiazolinone

DRAIN CLEANER
surfactants, fragrance, sodium hypochlorite, sodium hydroxide

AIR AND FABRIC FRESHENER
fragrance, sodium borate, trideceth-4

I know this list looks a little overwhelming. But knowing what's in the products you're using is the first step to a toxin-free home. Next, I'm going to teach you how to read all the labels on cleaning supplies—with good (but sometimes misleading) words like "organic" and "all natural" to yucky words like "xylene" and "formaldehyde." Once you come to recognize the ingredients to avoid, you'll feel much better about navigating the options.

How to Read Labels on Cleaning Products

Now that you've seen some of the common offenders, let's take a closer look at your cleaning products. If you're like me, standing in the cleaning products aisle trying to compare different items and what they promise can make your head swim! Not to mention trying to decipher all the listed chemicals on the labels. (Though not all chemicals are bad—for example, hydrogen peroxide is a chemical but it can also be used as a mouthwash and a safe disinfectant.) As you read through this chapter, it might help to grab one of your current products, such as a bottle of hand soap or dish soap, and use its label as a reference. From marketing slogans on the front that cheerily proclaim "All natural!" to the daunting list of ingredients on the back, I'll break down for you what they all mean so you can make the best choice.

Marketing Promises: "Organic" or "Natural" Products May Not Be What They Seem

If you've compared products at the store and chosen the one that had the words "nontoxic," "natural," or "green" on the label, I have good news and bad news for you. The good news is you most likely chose a better product than the ones that don't make these claims, and you've made the first step toward bringing home better choices. The bad news is that, unfortunately, none of the claims on bottles are checked or regulated. This is equal parts fascinating and maddening to me because I have fallen prey to the overpriced hype.

Here's what those marketing terms mean:

ORGANIC   A couple of different seals are under the "organic" umbrella: the USDA ORGANIC seal and an NSF INTERNATIONAL seal. Any products containing a seal have paid for and undergone third-party certification and should be trusted. If a company is found to have violated the labeling rules, they are fined.[1] In order for a product to bear the USDA ORGANIC seal, it must contain at least 95 percent organic ingredients. The product might also be labeled 100% ORGANIC, which means it has been produced or grown using only organic ingredients. When a product label contains the word "organic," you can also assume it's free of pesticides, synthetic or artificial ingredients, and genetically modified organisms (GMOs), and has not undergone irradiation.

An NSF INTERNATIONAL label on a product means the product has at least 70 percent organic ingredients.[2] Any company can claim that its product is organic or that it contains organic ingredients because there are no regulations on using the term "organic." If using organic products is important to you, read the labels and examine ingredients. Don't rely on just the product description. For instance, a product might tout "organic" in its description, but unless it has a seal, it may not be. This is why understanding what is in products is so important.

NATURAL   According to *Consumer Reports'* Greener Choices organization (Greener Choices.org), using the term "natural" on products and food has "no meaning." The term "natural" is not verified by a third-party source, "there are no consistent standards to ensure that the label means what it implies to consumers, . . . and each company can use its own definition, and definitions vary widely. Government agencies only provide guidance, not regulations, for companies using the 'natural' claim."[3] Bottom line: don't immediately trust a product just because it's labeled NATURAL. Go a step further and read the list of ingredients to determine if it's really safe for your home.

SYNTHETIC OR ARTIFICIAL FRAGRANCE   Most products have "fragrance" or "artificial fragrance" listed as an ingredient. If you see "fragrance" in a product's ingredients list, my advice is to steer clear. There is no regulation on fragrances, and fragrances pose a threat to your health and well-being simply because of the chemicals that go into, or might go into, them. I'll talk more about fragrances later in the book, but "synthetic" or "artificial" simply means they are human made. For instance, vanilla extract can be made from vanilla beans and alcohol or from artificial vanilla flavor. Which one would you buy? Something derived from the real thing will always be the better-tasting choice, and it's significantly better for you too!

NATURALLY DERIVED OR PLANT DERIVED "Naturally derived" generally means that the product has ingredients that occur in nature, and the term "plant derived" means that the product has ingredients derived from plants. (Very scientific, huh?) If you see this on a label, read the ingredients a little more closely. If a hand soap says "plant based" or "plant derived," that's a good thing! This means the soap isn't petroleum based.

NONTOXIC "Nontoxic" generally means it isn't going to kill you if you eat it, but it does not mean that you *should* eat it. This is another term that isn't regulated, so a company can make the claim, but the product may not have been tested or verified. If you use white vinegar to clean with and your child chugs some, he or she might have a tummy ache, but your child isn't going to need to go to the emergency room. Whereas if your child chugs a "nontoxic" cleaner you had on your counter and you aren't 100 percent sure of what its five ingredients are, you'll probably make a call to your pediatrician and/or Poison Control. Of course you want all your cleaners to be nontoxic, but it's still important to keep them away from children and pets. Just because something says it's nontoxic, that doesn't mean it really is.

VEGAN This might seem like an odd thing to list on a cleaning product since it simply means the item contains no animal products, but quite a few products out there do include animal by-products. It's difficult to figure out if a product is vegan because labels won't list "processed animal fat," and you might not know that "lipase" is derived from the pancreas of animals and used to make some laundry detergents more effective. If you aren't a vegan, this might not be a big deal to you—what's a little animal fat or pancreas in your detergent, right? (I'm kidding. Personally I think it's pretty gross.) But it's very important to vegans, and it's also just smart, as a consumer, to really know what's in the products in your home.

CRUELTY-FREE   "Cruelty-free" means that the product wasn't tested on animals in any way. This requires the product go through a certification process, and the company pays a small certification fee.[4] The product will then proudly display either a Leaping Bunny symbol (an international logo, verified by the Coalition for Consumer Information on Cosmetics),[5] a CRUELTY FREE bunny label (verified by PETA), or a BEAUTY WITHOUT BUNNIES symbol (verified by PETA). If buying cruelty-free products is important to you, do your research and/or contact a company about its products if you don't see a symbol on them.

GREEN   A product containing the term "green" is presumably environmentally safe and expected to have used safer manufacturing processes. This term is overused and highly marketed with no real proof or documentation necessary to employ it. Maybe you've heard the term "greenwashing," which refers to a company trying to make you think it's green or ecofriendly though it has no alternative business or ingredient practices. Just because a company says it's "green" doesn't make it so. It might be exploiting a niche in the market with just the right product at the right time.

NON-GMO   "Non-GMO" simply stands for "no genetically modified organisms." Companies proudly display this on food labels, but you will also see it on household and personal products.[6] If a product has undergone the third-party certification for this, it will bear a NON-GMO PROJECT seal with a butterfly on a blade of grass. This certification is important, especially with food, because it ensures the product hasn't been genetically tampered with in any way or fed products that have been genetically altered. According to the Non-GMO Project, there is evidence that GMOs cause health and environmental damage. The United States does not currently require GM ingredients be labeled as such on products, but more than sixty other countries do.[7] Consumers are taking matters into their own hands and choosing to opt out of GMOs.

Quite a few small "green" companies have been bought by large companies that make some unsafe products. I've listed a few here. (It should also be noted that when a company is purchased by another company, it doesn't mean the buying company has taken over production.)

MRS. MEYER'S CLEAN DAY
is now owned by SC Johnson

SEVENTH GENERATION
is now owned by Unilever

TOM'S OF MAINE
is now owned by Colgate-Palmolive

AVEENO
is now owned by Johnson & Johnson

BURT'S BEES
is now owned by Clorox

ANNIE'S HOMEGROWN
AND LÄRABAR
are now owned by General Mills

I've found that these companies aren't what they used to be or what I thought they were. I use a couple of Seventh Generation products but have found replacements for my other favorites. It's not worth the risk when there are other products out there that are 100 percent safe. If the same company that makes a known toxic cleaning spray also makes a "natural" bathroom cleaning spray, I'm a wee bit skeptical of the "natural" claim. Throughout the book, I'll point to companies and brands that I've found make the best, safest cleaning products. (You can also find them listed in the appendix on page 195.)

CERTIFIED B CORPORATION This seal shows consumers that the company takes interest in the well-being of its workers, its community, and the environment. This is reflected in the products it uses, its shipping methods, its policies, and other factors. In order to bear this seal, a company must have a verified score of 80 points out of 200.[8] This qualification is more about business and environmental practices than what's in the products the company carries. B Corporation certification is definitely a good thing, but with such a large range of points, I find it more useful as a starting point to determine if a company's products are safe to use.

The Ingredients Label

You can read and research until you're so confused that you aren't even sure what's true anymore (ask me how I know!), but the easiest thing to do is to start with safe products and build from there. If you still want to research each and every ingredient on a label, you might think twice when you hear this: the National Institute for Occupational Safety and Health researched almost 3,000 ingredients already used in homes and found that 778 ingredients could be acutely toxic to the human body, 314 can cause biological mutation, 218 can cause reproductive complications, and 146 can cause tumors.[9] Additionally, EWG reports that throughout the last thirty years, the voluntary program Cosmetic Ingredient Review (CIR)—an ingredients assessment process funded primarily by trade associations—has reviewed only "about 11% of the ingredients in products, or 1,400 out of what FDA estimates is a total of 12,500 ingredients in personal care products."[10] With the current standards in place, companies can use any ingredients with no standards or requirements for safety required.

That information is enough for me to say, "Throw everything away and just use soap and water." Depending on where you're starting from, that might be you. If you've already started to eliminate chemicals and toxic products, hooray! You've probably already figured out some good swaps in your home. Regardless of your journey, here are just a handful of the chemicals you might find in your household products:

AMMONIA   Naturally occurring, ammonia is found in the environment as a gas. It's in the earth, air, water, and plants, and it's produced by humans after we eat foods containing protein—our bodies convert ammonia into urea. Ammonium hydroxide is what is found in cleaners and sold as a stand-alone cleaning product.[11]

Ammonia is hazardous right out of the container as a respiratory irritant and can cause burns to the skin and organ damage.[12] Yet you can use it in your home straight out of the bottle. It's also in a lot of window cleaners, but it's best to steer clear of these and any products that list "ammonia" or "ammonium hydroxide" as an ingredient.

ANTIMICROBIALS AND ANTIBACTERIALS   At first glance, these products— often antimicrobial soaps and hand sanitizers—look like a healthy choice for keeping your family safe from germs, but they are known endocrine disruptors and are bad for the environment. An added and very real concern is that the chemicals used in antibacterials and antimicrobials actually cause germs to mutate and become anti-biotic resistant. The FDA banned triclosan, used in soaps, detergents, toothpastes, and other products, in September 2016 (effective September 2017) due to superbug concerns, but that doesn't mean triclosan is gone.[13] Stay away from any items that make an antibacterial or antimicrobial claim.

BENZENE   Benzene is a sweet-smelling, colorless chemical derived from crude oil, natural gas, or coal. It's also found in volcanoes and forest fires. The list of side effects and health issues is long, but what's most important to know is that exposure to ben-zene can cause the body's blood cells to not work correctly, can cause immediate dizziness, and is considered to be a carcinogen.[14] Benzene can be found in many detergents and household cleaners.

BLEACH—SODIUM HYPOCHLORITE   Sodium hypochlorite is the primary ingredient found in bleach as well as a disinfectant found in other cleaners. While bleach is dangerous on its own, it can be deadly when combined with household cleaners like ammonia, vinegar, toilet bowl cleaners, drain cleaners, and spray cleaners. Even water mixed with bleach can be dangerous.[15]

Bleach is considered an irritant to skin, tissues, and the respiratory system. While bleach does what it says it will do—it's an effective cleaning agent—the risks outweigh the gains.

1,4-DIOXANE   Found in many laundry products and cleaning solutions, and used to make a solution foamy, this is an ingredient to steer clear of. Here's the warning on 1,4-dioxane from the US Environmental Protection Agency (EPA): "Likely to be carcinogenic to humans by all routes of exposure . . . Short-term exposure may cause eye, nose, and throat irritation; long-term exposure may cause kidney and liver damage . . . It is a by-product present in many goods, including paint strippers, dyes, greases, antifreeze, and aircraft deicing fluids, and in some consumer products (deodorants, shampoos, and cosmetics)."[16] According to EWG's Skin Deep database, it's in at least 46 percent of personal care products.[17] You typically won't find it listed on labels because it's actually a by-product of a combination of chemicals.

Where will you find 1,4-dioxane? Any product that gets sudsy or foamy—soaps and shampoos are where you'll find it most often. Look for these ingredients: PEG compounds, polysorbate, and ingredients ending in "xynol" and "eth"— nonoxynol and sodium laureth sulfate are examples.

FORMALDEHYDE   Formaldehyde is found in manufactured wood products such as oriented strand board (OSB), plywood, medium-density fiberboard (MDF), and particleboard, which are used in building materials and furniture, including kitchen cabinets, desks, bookshelves, and beds. Although formaldehyde emissions from wood products reduce over time, there are many other invisible sources in the home. It is also added to paints, coatings, plastic products, pesticides, cosmetics, adhesives, glues, resins, synthetic fabrics, mattress ticking, permanent-press bedding, leather goods, clothing, and drapes. Plus, formaldehyde is a combustion by-product of cigarette smoke and unvented, fuel-burning appliances, like gas stoves and space heaters.

The highest levels of airborne formaldehyde have been detected in indoor air, where it's released from various building materials and home furnishings. One survey reported formaldehyde levels ranging from 0.10 to 3.68 parts per million (ppm) in homes. Higher levels have been found in newly manufactured or mobile homes than in older conventional homes.

Acute formaldehyde exposure via inhalation results in eye, nose, and throat irritation; affects the nasal cavity; and may produce coughing, wheezing, chest pains, and bronchitis.[18]

Pay attention to clothing labels and avoid "easy care" fabrics: permanent-press, anticling, antistatic, antiwrinkle, and antishrink (especially shrink-proof wool), stain-resistant (especially for suede and chamois), mildew-resistant, waterproof, perspiration-proof, moth-proof, and color-fast. In order to meet these qualifications, these fabrics are often treated with urea-formaldehyde resins.[19] You won't find this listed on the fabrics, making it even more tricky.

In 2009, TSA officers found that their new uniforms, the fabric of which was laced with formaldehyde, were contributing to rashes, skin irritations, runny or bloody noses, light-headedness, red eyes, and swollen and cracked lips.[20] Formaldehyde is also associated with more severe health issues.[21] For example, it could cause nervous system damage by its ability to react with and form cross-links with proteins, DNA, and unsaturated fatty acids. These same mechanisms could cause damage to virtually any cell in the body since all cells contain these substances. Formaldehyde can react with nerve proteins (neuroamines) and nerve transmitters (catecholamines), which could impair normal nervous system function and cause endocrine disruption.

NONYLPHENOL ETHOXYLATE (NPE)   Nonylphenol ethoxylate is a surfactant in many cleaning products. While it's banned in both Europe and Canada due to safety concerns and its health effects, it's still prevalent in the United States.

NPE disrupts the endocrine system as well as negatively affects both physical function and fetal development. An endocrine disruptor is a chemical that disrupts or changes the hormonal system.[22] These changes can happen in utero or to anyone, and the exposure can occur via a use of simple chemicals, plastics, or fragrances. Numerous systems in the body can be compromised by exposure to this chemical, including the immune system, nervous system, kidneys, heart, and liver. Infants and children are especially sensitive to NPE.

PARABEN   Paraben is used in personal care products, like body washes, shampoos, conditioners, lotions, toothpastes, deodorants, and makeup. Known endocrine disruptors, parabens have been linked to cancer as well as reproductive and developmental toxicity.[23] Look carefully at labels, because "paraben" might not be easily seen on the label; there might instead be a word containing "paraben," like "methylparaben" or "butylparaben." Any ingredient with "paraben" in its name is considered a paraben and should be avoided.

PHENOL   From the Human Metabolome Database: "Phenol is a toxic, colorless crystalline solid with a sweet tarry odor that resembles a hospital smell. It is commonly used as an antiseptic and disinfectant. It is active against a wide range of microorganisms, including some fungi and viruses, but is only slowly effective against spores."[24]

Phenol is a very common chemical and is regularly found in the following products: cold capsules, cough syrups, bronchial mists, Chloraseptic throat sprays, decongestants, aspirin, aftershaves, deodorants, feminine powders and sprays, cosmetics, hair sprays, hair-setting lotions, lice shampoos, acne medications, mouthwashes, antiseptics, anti-itching lotions, calamine lotion, hand lotions, sunscreens, lip balms, solvents, detergents, air fresheners, furniture polishes, all-purpose cleaners, disinfectant cleaners, aerosol disinfectants, and insecticides.

Phenol is an extremely caustic chemical that burns the skin in high concentrations. A product may have only a small amount of phenol in it, producing little or no side effect, but this ingredient should still be avoided because of the potential harm it could do. Absorption of phenol through the lungs or skin can cause central nervous system damage, pneumonia, respiratory tract infection, heart-rate irregularities, skin irritation, kidney and liver damage, numbness, or vomiting, and it can be fatal.[25] Small amounts of phenol have been fine for some people but toxic to others. This is one of those cases where I'd rather be on the safe side and stay away from products that list phenol as one of the ingredients.

PHOSPHATE   A phosphate is a chemical compound that contains both phosphorus and oxygen. Occurring naturally, phosphates are prevalent in many dish soaps, detergents, and household cleaners. They work by dissolving particles of dirt as well as removing stains by softening the water, causing suds to form. This poses harm to the environment because phosphates remain active even after wastewater facilities chemically treat water. Phosphates also encourage algae growth, which negatively affects marine and plant life as well as creates dead zones in bodies of water—areas depleted of oxygen.

Phosphates are also found in foods, like cured meats and cheeses, and sodas. They act as a preservative, so one would think they're harmless. Right? Wrong. According to a study published in the journal *EMBO Molecular Medicine,* there's a correlation between phosphates and heart disease, kidney disease, and high blood pressure, where phosphates were found to up the production of a hormone that causes these diseases.[26] Be on the lookout for phosphates in your cleaning products *and* in your food!

PHTHALATE   Phthalates can cause birth defects, harm the reproductive and endocrine systems, and promote cancer. You'll find phthalates in perfumes, synthetic or "fake" fragrances, shampoos and conditioners, makeup, nail polishes, and lotions. Phthalates are unregulated and often added to fragrances—look for cosmetics and products labeled PHTHALATE-FREE.[27]

SODIUM LAURYL SULFATE, SODIUM LAURETH SULFATE, AND AMMONIUM LAUREL SULFATE   Sodium lauryl sulfate (SLS), sodium laureth sulfate (SLES), and ammonium laurel sulfate (ALS) are very common ingredients in many cleaning supplies. They add foaming qualities to detergents as well as act as surfactants and emulsifiers. Surfactants are substances that, when added to a liquid, reduce surface tension, allowing, say, a detergent to penetrate a fabric. Emulsifiers lift and separate oils and fats, allowing them to be rinsed away.

Sulfates are mainly linked to skin and eye irritation, but they are also associated with endocrine disruption and cellular changes, with some lower concern for ecotoxicology.[28]

SYNTHETIC, OR ARTIFICIAL, FRAGRANCE—PARFUM, PERFUME   Synthetic fragrances consist of various chemicals that combine to produce scents. The vast majority of synthetic fragrances are made from petroleum and other toxic chemicals. Many cleaning supplies and detergents contain synthetic fragrances to appeal to the consumer.

These chemicals not only irritate the senses but are also linked to cancer, birth defects, central nervous system disorders, and allergic reactions. Just do a quick internet search of "harmful fragrance" and you'll unearth all sorts of information, warnings, and statistics that point to just how dangerous fragrance is. You'll see it called the new secondhand smoke, a carcinogen, a cancer causer, an endocrine disruptor, and the most common cause of asthma attacks, to name a few.

But how did we get here? Has fragrance always been bad? Interestingly, up until the 1970s and 1980s most perfumes/parfums were made from natural sources, like herbs, flowers, and citrus. Rose perfume had distilled rose petals in it. Lemon furniture polish had lemon oil in it. Fast-forward to today, and according to EWG, there are up to fourteen hidden ingredients in any given "fragrance."[29]

This means that if a company has ten different fragrances that make up their "fresh scent," all they need to include in the ingredients list is "fragrance." The Fair Packaging and Labeling Act of 1967 was intended to make sure that consumers knew what they were purchasing and that labels weren't deceptive or misleading.[30] Yet this act also allowed companies to keep their fragrances secret so no one else could replicate them. Through the years this has become the loophole allowing fragrances to be an entity in and of themselves. Since companies don't have to disclose what a fragrance really is, we consumers don't know what chemicals are in their products, and in turn, we cannot determine the full effects of using those products. Taking a hard pass on any product that contains fragrance means that you'll eliminate that risk from your home.[31]

XYLENE   Xylene comes in three forms, called isomers (ortho-, meta-, and para-xylene), and is a colorless, sweet-smelling, and highly flammable liquid that occurs naturally in petroleum and coal tar. It is used as a solvent, a cleaning agent, and a paint thinner.[32]

Short-term exposure to high levels of xylene can cause irritation of the skin, eyes, nose, and throat; difficulty in breathing; impaired function of the lungs; delayed response to a visual stimulus; impaired memory; stomach discomfort; and possible changes in the liver and kidneys. Both short- and long-term exposure to high concentrations of xylene can also cause a number of effects on the nervous system, such as headaches, lack of muscle coordination, dizziness, confusion, and changes in one's sense of balance.[33]

All this may be information overload, but I hope you can refer to this list as you purchase new cleaning products and assess the ones you already have. The more you know, the better prepared you are to keep your home safe.

CHAPTER 3

The Toxic Ten and Whole Home Swaps

HAVE YOU HEARD OF THE DIRTY DOZEN PRODUCE LIST? IT RANKS THE TWELVE MOST pesticide-laden fruits and vegetables tested by the Environmental Working Group (EWG) for residue.[1] The recommendation is that you should always buy this produce as organic or just don't buy these items at all. I don't have a problem staying away from sweet bell peppers, but everything else on the list is a favorite in our home, so we make the switch to organic.

Just like you might choose to avoid the most pesticide-riddled fruits and vegetables, you can also swap out the ten most toxic household products—I call them my Toxic Ten. I'm guessing that some of these products are your favorites. What's more, you might think you're already using a safe alternative. This was me! I thought I'd found safe alternatives for so many of my former favorite conventional products because they were labeled NATURAL or ECOFRIENDLY. You guessed it: once I did the research, I found these products rated just as badly as the products that weren't claiming to do anything but clean. While you keep reading I'm going to go breathe into a paper bag and calm down—I'm still upset about it.

When I tell you what the worst offenders are in your home, I'm not going to just drop that information on you and walk away. I'll give you some solutions, including products you can make yourself as well as brands and alternatives you can trust. The whole-home swaps I suggest will be cheap, easy to find, and quick to put together. This is important, because in order to make a swap, you have to have a game plan, and the solution has to be just as good or better than the original. Think for a minute about the food analogy. If strawberries are your favorite fruit and you eat them every day but see that they rank the highest for pesticide residue, what do you do? Look for organic strawberries the next time you're at the store. That can get expensive, so one solution I've found is to buy frozen organic strawberries in bulk at my favorite warehouse store and use those for smoothies, then buy the fresh organic strawberries when they're on sale or at a promo price. You can follow the same easy practice with your cleaning supplies. And by swapping out toxic products for easy solutions, you'll find you save money and feel so much better about what you're using in your home.

The Toxic Ten

1 PESTICIDES seem logical, but I think we're so accustomed to using pesticides and various chemical treatments on our homes and lawns that this is an area that goes unnoticed. Even if you don't apply the pesticide yourself, you can still bring it into your home, and pets and kids are exposed to it readily in parks and in your neighborhood. There are hidden pesticides in fabrics, on and in foods, in insect repellants, and in pet insect treatments. Just when you think you're doing pretty good, this bomb is dropped—pesticide residue is everywhere.

swap

First, if you have kids in school, ask to be informed when the school grounds or buildings are being treated so you can take precautions with your children if they're sensitive or if you just don't want them to be exposed or bring the residue home on their shoes. With my kids' schools, I get an email the day before a "treatment," and I don't keep the kids out of school, but I might clean off the bottoms of their shoes. Plus, we won't go to the playground that evening.

Next, if you use a lawn-care service, ask if they have organic options—many companies are adding alternatives. If your service doesn't, look for one that uses natural or organic products instead of synthetic chemicals. Implement lawn-care methods that make the soil healthier.[2] Try adding compost and alfalfa meal in lieu of fertilizer as you build up the soil over time, instead of chemically treating the grass and weeds. This slow process eventually leads to drought-resistant grass and a much healthier lawn. A handful of companies offer this service nationwide. NaturaLawn is the largest network of organic lawn-care providers in the United States.

Don't use insect repellents with DEET; instead opt for insect sprays that use picaridin and IR3535, both at 20 percent concentration (Aunt Fannie's brand makes cleaning and pest control products). With the Zika virus warnings, it's important to protect yourself and your family from mosquitos carrying diseases. EWG recommends wearing clothing that covers your arms and legs if possible, and use insect repellant that works.[3] When you come inside, shower to remove any residue.

Avoid pesticides for your pets, especially flea and tick collars. Instead use a product like Revolution, which is a once-a-month treatment. I was surprised when my holistic veterinarian recommended this for our dog, but she said that the risk of infestation isn't worth taking.

Look for organic bedding. Organic bedding is typically 100 percent cotton, and the cotton isn't treated with pesticides. It's practically impossible to buy all organic clothing, so I recommend always washing clothing before wearing it to effectively remove any chemical residue.

LAUNDRY DETERGENT washes out of clothing and smells divine, right? But that smell—the artificial fragrance—is toxic and can seep into the skin. I'm guessing you or someone you know has had to switch detergents after getting a rash or breaking out. That reaction can be from the ingredients, the fragrance, or the "optical brighteners"—synthetic chemicals used to make your clothing appear bright, white, and clean. The fragrance in laundry detergent is formulated to embed in the fibers so it stays with you, but that chemical fragrance is what is particularly harmful to your body and the environment.

Unfortunately you can't just grab a "free and clear" detergent, because that probably has artificial fragrances too—to cover up the product's own fragrance and to simulate it being unscented. Isn't that horrible? That's why people with sensitive skin or eczema can still have irritation with fragrance-free laundry products.

Look for a laundry detergent made with naturally derived, plant-based ingredients, and if it's scented, make sure it uses pure essential oils, not a synthetically sourced scent. Or make your own! On page 165 I'll share with you my favorite DIY laundry detergent recipe. If you're looking for alternatives, I love Molly's Suds Laundry Detergent, and they make the version I sell in my Clean Mama online shop too (CleanMamaHome.net). A couple of other safe recommendations are Better Life and Branch Basics Concentrate.

FABRIC SOFTENER AND DRYER SHEETS make your laundry soft and static-free, but at what cost? Fabric softeners have the same ingredient issues as laundry detergents, plus most conventional fabric softeners are not only toxic but also coat the fibers of fabrics, making items harder to clean because the softener builds up on them. Dryer sheets are even worse. A study out of the University of Washington showed that there are twenty-five volatile organic compounds (VOCs) in dryer sheets, seven hazardous air pollutants, and two known carcinogens.[4] Since we know carcinogens cause cancer, it's just smart to stay away from conventional dryer sheets. Consider this too: the exhaust from your dryer vent with a dryer sheet is even harmful to the environment as a pollutant.[5] That exposure is very minimal compared to what ends up on your clothing, but I'll take a little pant leg static every day of the week. The good news is there are alternatives!

I love wool dryer balls. They last almost forever (at least one thousand loads), the wool helps reduce static, and they can be custom-scented with your favorite essential oils (see pages 53 and 136). You can also put a little vinegar on them and use them in the wash, just as you would use a liquid fabric softener. See the appendix for where to purchase them.

ANTIBACTERIAL SOAP most likely includes triclosan, which is added to all sorts of things, including toothpastes and body washes. Triclosan was banned in the United States in September 2016 (effective September 2017) because of superbug concerns, but it's still found on ingredients lists in this country. Studies have shown a link between antibiotic resistance and antibacterial products. My recommendation is to use plain old soap and water. According to the FDA, a good hand washing with plain soap removes most germs and bacteria just as well as a product that claims to be antibacterial.[6]

Look for soap without any "antibacterial" claims, and make sure it doesn't have triclosan or fragrance in its ingredients. Find a brand that contains essential oils, is plant (not petroleum) derived, and doesn't have parabens. My absolute favorites? EO and Everyone—both lines are made by the same company.

HAND SANITIZER isn't always a bad product. In fact, I have a couple on hand for when we aren't near soap and water—but make sure that any hand sanitizer you purchase doesn't have triclosan, artificial fragrance, and/or synthetic ingredients. Those ingredients outweigh the benefits of a quick hand washing. You might also find parabens and phthalates lurking in your beloved hand sanitizer.

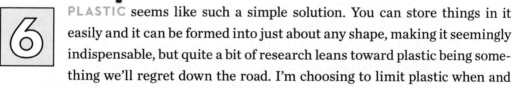

EO brand carries a small package of hand wipes and a spray. I keep both in my purse. I also like Dr. Bronner's hand sanitizer spray—the lavender is lovely. These favorites include ingredients such as rubbing alcohol, glycerin, and essential oil. You can also make one of the recipes I provide later in the book—it's surprisingly simple (see pages 125 and 126).

PLASTIC seems like such a simple solution. You can store things in it easily and it can be formed into just about any shape, making it seemingly indispensable, but quite a bit of research leans toward plastic being something we'll regret down the road. I'm choosing to limit plastic when and where I can. One concern about plastic is the endocrine-disrupting chemicals—bisphenol A (BPA) and other polycarbonate plastics as well as phthalates (added for pliability). We know that BPA is harmful in food products, but it can still be found in unexpected places, like receipts, toilet paper, canned foods, plastic wrap, and disposable kitchenware, like plates, cups, and utensils.[7]

Avoid plastic whenever possible, including plastic drinking straws, plastic wrap, water bottles, shopping bags, toys, home storage solutions, and food storage containers (which we'll discuss in more detail next).

If you choose to keep plastics in your kitchen, don't microwave food in them (the heat of the microwave will leach the chemicals into your food), and look for the numbers 2, 4, and/or 5 on the bottom, as they are safer. Completely avoid 3, 6, and 7 for food or beverage storage. Recycle plastics whenever possible.

There are so many alternatives to plastic these days. Some simple swaps to make are milk packaged in paper or glass containers; fun paper or metal straws instead of plastic; and washable, paper, or waxed-paper varieties of sandwich or snack bags.

If you use plastic wrap to keep all kinds of foods fresh, consider switching to an alternative like Bee's Wrap.[8] It's cotton (washable and reusable) that has been coated with beeswax, organic jojoba oil, and tree resin. Other alternatives for bowl covers are made from fabric or oilcloth, which can be found online and even on Etsy, or you can look for a DIY version online and make your own.

Just doing a search for reusable water bottles will give you hundreds of options—and even better, they're so stylish, they've become a fashion statement. While writing this book, I switched out our BPA-free plastic water bottles for stainless steel. My favorite is the Yeti for smoothies—my husband and I each have one—and I have a stash of S'ip by S'well water bottles for the kids. They love that their water stays cold all day, and I love that nothing's seeping into their water while it waits for them in their lunch box.

There are also a lot of practical, stylish options for reusable grocery bags. Invest in some, then stash them in your purse and your car so you always have one ready when you make a last-minute trip to the store. Look for bags that can be washed—if they're holding your raw meat, even though it's packaged, you're going to want to wash that bag later! I use small, foldable grocery bags that fit into a little pocket or my purse; otherwise, I would probably forget them at home. Also, reusable mesh bags are perfect for fruits and veggies, and they help you avoid those plastic produce bags (that take five minutes to open). I like the Flip & Tumble brand; they have color-coded tabs for different types of produce, and they're thin and washable with an easy-to-use drawstring.

Opt for wood or natural toys for kids. Not only will these toys last longer; kids love playing with them too. Try the Hape brand, which has so many options, from play kitchens to trucks to puzzles.

Look for natural home storage solutions when possible, like baskets made from fabric or wicker or wire instead of plastic or acrylic.

$\boxed{7}$ FOOD STORAGE SOLUTIONS are something I encourage you to completely swap out for non-plastic alternatives. Even though there are a lot of warnings now about BPA in plastics, and you may find it difficult to locate products made with BPA (since it was banned in 2012 from baby bottles and sippy cups[9]), plastic still isn't the most desirable material for food storage, especially long-term food storage. It still has phthalates you want to avoid and other chemicals, such as other forms of bisphenol. For example, canned foods still might contain a material with BPA, so look for canned goods labeled BPA-FREE.

For lunches and on-the-go storage, I recommend 100 percent stainless steel. It will last forever and takes the breakable factor out of the equation. For storing leftovers at home, glass containers are a good choice. I especially like using glass canning jars to store food and/or salads. (I don't send glass to school with the kids.) There are many options on the market in every size and configuration. Do a quick search on the internet, and you'll find hundreds of thousands of options. I use LunchBots Trio II stainless-steel food containers for the kids' lunches and ECOlunchbox.

AIR FRESHENERS—certainly the most conventional ones—are toxic for you because of the phenols, benzene, and formaldehyde present in the fragrance. Air fresheners can cause respiratory issues and have been linked to neurological problems and cancer while presenting many other potential problems, the least of which are asthma and allergies.[10]

Start using diffusers with pure essential oils instead of plug-ins. (See the appendix on page 198 for a list of some good brands.) Diffusing lavender can offer a calming effect, while tea tree oil is cleansing.

If you have an area of the home that smells damp or musty, get to the bottom of why it's musty, then get a dehumidifier or put a box of baking soda in place to absorb the odors. Have a lingering kitchen smell? Place a small bowl of white vinegar in the vicinity of the smell and let it sit for twelve to twenty-four hours; it will absorb the odor. Dump white vinegar down your sink, and your sink will benefit from its natural disinfecting qualities.

DISHWASHER DETERGENT gets your dishes clean, but in the process it often washes your plates and silverware with a whole host of chemicals, including bleach, fragrance, sodium hypochlorite, anti-foaming agents, and phosphates. Yes, the ingredients should be thoroughly washed down the drain, but they are still getting into the water system, and it's not hard to believe that some residue remains on the dishes.

Look for a dishwasher detergent without any of the ingredients I just listed, plus one that is fragrance-free. Some examples include Grab Green Fragrance-Free Dishwashing Detergent Pods, Seventh Generation Free and Clear Dishwashing Detergent Packs, Biokleen Automatic Dish Powder, and Better Life Dishwasher Gel. You can also make your own tablets with my recipe on page 101. DIYing dish detergent is difficult for quite a few reasons—everyone's dishwasher works differently, everyone has different hot-water temperatures, and then there's hard water, soft water, and whether you have a water softener. All of this works together to make a homemade dishwasher tablet a little difficult. But experiment with this recipe and see what works for you. Using a DIY version will give you peace of mind as you eat your dinner without any second-guessing.

HAND SOAP AND DISH SOAP can be tricky. Earlier I told you that while I was doing my research I changed my hand soap and dish soap. I thought I had picked good and safe alternatives, but I fell into the trap of buying a soap based on the company's claims of being "natural." When I saw on EWG.org that they contain ingredients that can cause skin irritation and allergies and contain artificial fragrances, I tossed them and looked for better alternatives.

swap Unfortunately, safe alternatives in the hand and dish soap realm are hard to come by. Brands I recommend are EO, Everyone, Rebel Green, and Better Life. However, the best alternative I've found is to make my own. Here's an easy and safe hand soap swap: get a soap dispenser with a foaming pump—a quick search on the internet will turn up quite a few options (if you look for plastic ones, make sure they're BPA-free)—fill it with water, add a squirt of liquid castile soap, shake it up, and you have a safe foaming soap that probably costs two cents per container. See pages 99 and 100 for more recipes, and try any essential oil combination you like to add fun, safe scents.

Quick temperature check: How are you feeling about all this information? Frustrated, mad, determined, or overwhelmed? It's understandable. Me? I'm feeling hopeful. We've identified the primary troublemakers as well as easy ideas for better cleaning solutions. Let's keep going to get to the bottom of all the product misinformation and to find more quick changes you can put into place right now. Then we'll move on to realistic swaps for every area of your home.

CHAPTER 4

The Secret to Going Organic Without Spending a Fortune

N THE LAST FEW CHAPTERS, WE DOVE DEEP INTO WHY SO MANY OF THE PRODUCTS WE bring into our home are dangerous and toxic. Now that you know what the problem is, what can you do to fix it? I'm glad you asked, because just as important as getting rid of bad products is bringing good choices into your home moving forward. Purchasing a safe cleaning spray and choosing a mattress free of formaldehyde will make your home safer. It's those lasting changes and habits that will make the real difference.

One lasting change you can make is to switch to buying organic products. I know, organic can equal expensive. Anyone who shops at a store that sells primarily organic food knows what I'm talking about. Everything looks so fresh and healthy, and the next thing you know, you've spent your paycheck on that cart of food! We're not going to do that with our home care products. I'll show you how you can actually *save* money by switching to organic, natural products. Instead of a cabinet bursting with different cleaning products, you'll have a curated handful of products that have multiple uses and are inexpensive to purchase. By choosing multipurpose products, you eliminate extras and create your own "concentrates" and cleaning solutions. And if figuring out how to make your own cleaning and homecare products feels a step too far for you, that's not a problem. I'll provide examples in later chapters of many safe product recommendations as well.

Let's start with the very basics. The secret to going organic without spending a fortune? Keep it *simple*. Plant-based, chemical-free, fragrance-free, natural, and organic solutions are probably already in your home. Better yet, these items can kill bacteria and germs, get rid of dust and grime, and keep your home safe. To clean your entire house organically you really only need something that cleans (soap and/or vinegar); something that scrubs, an abrasive (baking soda); and something to disinfect (hydrogen peroxide). You can grab all three ingredients for around fifteen dollars and they will last you months. Talk about cost effective!

We'll branch out later in the book into other ingredients, uses, and wonderfully effective recipes, but starting with the basics is helpful for many reasons—the most important is just seeing what you *can* clean with less. Do you need to purchase 100 percent certified organic baking soda to safely scrub your sink? No. Baking soda is an organic, naturally occurring compound. You can choose to purchase the orange box or another. There are plenty of certified-organic vinegars and baking sodas out there, but if you use the non-organic varieties (I do!), you are still cleaning "organically"—it just isn't considered "certified organic."

So how can you clean your whole home organically and naturally? With simply four products: soap, white vinegar, baking soda, and hydrogen peroxide.

I hope the quick reference chart on the following page shows that you don't need a new product for each and every surface of your home. A separate bathroom cleaner for your shower, toilet, counter, and floor simply isn't necessary, because each surface does *not* need a different chemical or solution. Each plastic bottle and its contents run the risk of harming your family, and each plastic bottle is meant to last and will sit empty in a landfill indefinitely. What's more, Americans spend around fifty dollars a month on household and cleaning supplies—that's a lot![1] Let's put our money toward products that won't hurt us and figure out how we can make the process simple and sustainable at the same time.

Minimizing what you have in your home will help you breathe easier, literally and figuratively. And it simplifies cleaning. For example, if that counter is bugging you and you want to clean it, just grab an empty spray bottle, fill it with water and add a drop or two of dish soap. Give it a shake, spray the mixture liberally on the counter, and wipe it clean. If you aren't a DIYer, I have plenty of solutions for you too. There are options on the market that will still keep the supplies to a minimum from companies that keep your health and well-being at the forefront of their mission.

Here's a quick reference chart of what you can clean with just the basics. See page 77 for specific recipes and ratios.

Counters—vinegar and water or soap and water (note: do not use vinegar on marble or granite)

Toilets—vinegar and water on surfaces and baking soda and soap in the bowl

Appliances—vinegar and water

Hydrogen Peroxide—Any hard surface that needs to be disinfected.

Floors—soap and water

Baseboards and walls—soap and water

Carpet—vinegar and water

Dust—dusting wand, cloth, or vacuum

CHAPTER 5

The Whole Home Detox Pantry

THE EASIEST WAY TO START CLEANING NATURALLY IS TO PUT TOGETHER A CUSTOM-ized Whole Home Detox Pantry. I'm going to indicate which ingredients you should keep in your pantry as well as the best tools to keep on hand to make cleaning a breeze. The ingredients will get you through the entire detox process. I also will introduce each product so you know exactly what it is and how to use it. I hope this gets you excited about using these products in your home. Knowing what they can do will help you to maximize their effectiveness and minimize your effort at the same time. Simplification at its best!

First Things First: Create Space for the Whole Home Detox Pantry

In the next section is a list of twelve ingredients that will make up your new pantry. All of these ingredients can be purchased for under thirty dollars and will most likely last two to three months, if not more. After that, I'll show you the seven best cleaning tools to also keep in your pantry so that you'll be ready to go!

To start, find a place to keep the ingredients. I suggest devoting something you already have—a basket, a bin, or a cleared-off shelf—for your pantry supplies. Having everything together in one place, easily accessible, simplifies your cleaning. And by arming yourself with products that will safely and effectively clean your home, you'll be less likely to grab that old cleaner you know is bad for your health.

Essentials for the Whole Home Detox Pantry

1. *Hydrogen peroxide:* Hydrogen peroxide is unstable when it comes into contact with light so you need to keep it in its original brown bottle. If it spills onto colored clothing, carpet, towels, etc., it will bleach the fibers. It also is a weak acid, so *do not* use it on stone (granite, marble, etc.), as it will etch the surface over time.

   USES FOR HYDROGEN PEROXIDE:

   - Use straight out of the bottle if you're pretreating a stain (on white clothing). If it's a teeny, tiny stain, use a cotton swab to zero in on the stain.

   - Mix about 1 teaspoon hydrogen peroxide with 1 tablespoon or so baking soda for a cleaning paste, scrub the surface, and rinse clean. This works well for icky grout as well as sinks, especially for deep cleaning the kitchen sink and garbage disposal. If you have a larger surface area to clean (like a tiled shower floor) you can sprinkle the surface with baking soda, spray it thoroughly with hydrogen peroxide, and use a scrub brush to scrub, scrub, scrub away stains and grime.

   - My favorite method? Simply put a sprayer on the hydrogen peroxide brown bottle, spray straight hydrogen peroxide onto a surface that needs disinfection, let it sit, then rinse it clean. If you want to give germs the one-two punch, spray a surface with hydrogen peroxide and follow that with white vinegar sprayed from a separate bottle. Let it sit and rinse it clean. This is a very potent combination, and the two ingredients should *never* be combined in a container—always keep them separate.

2. *Soap:* My preference is castile soap, which is a natural, vegetable-based product made primarily of coconut and olive oils. Available in bar or liquid form, castile soap is simply soap made from naturally found and sourced ingredients. The Dr. Bronner's brand is widely available and comes in a variety of scents, like almond, citrus, and tea tree, as well as an unscented baby version. As a sidenote, the bar (not the liquid) baby soap contains sodium hydroxide (an ingredient I warn against using) before saponification (the finished soap product), but upon saponification the sodium hydroxide is no longer present. Castile soap is affordable, extremely concentrated, natural, and gentle, and it cleans beautifully! It's a powerhouse of a multipurpose cleaner, and it's so safe that you can use it to clean fruit and vegetables, and to brush your teeth. One word of caution: castile soap and vinegar don't mix. The acid in the vinegar when combined with the castile makes a sludge. This solution would still be effective, but it's going to look a little gross.

In lieu of castile, look for any vegetable-based (not petroleum-based) dish soap, making sure it has no antibacterial or antimicrobial claims. Double-check the ingredient list too for "triclosan" or "triclocarban" to make triple sure you have a safe choice in your hands. If you go the route of dish soap, also look for one without fragrance. Essential oils are fine, but any added fragrance is a no-no.

3. *White vinegar:* You know the stuff. Plain distilled white vinegar. You can get a gallon or so of it at a warehouse store for less than three dollars or you can find it at the grocery store by the other vinegars. You can even purchase organic white vinegar if you prefer. It's a wonderful, multipurpose cleaner. I use it in the laundry

room as a fabric softener and a deodorizer, but it works just as well as a cleaner and a disinfectant.

But what about that pickle smell?! I definitely sing the praises of distilled white vinegar now, but—true story—I put off using it for years because I hate that pickle smell. I know many people feel the same. Combined with the right essential oils and plenty of water, it's not so bad, and that smell completely dissipates once it's dry. Really, it does!

4. *Baking soda:* The orange box in your pantry or baking cupboard? That little box is a powerhouse. You can use it to scrub away tough stains and shine your sinks, showers, and tubs. You can also use it to deodorize or freshen up everything from a refrigerator to a mattress to a carpet. Your Whole Home Detox Pantry should always have a box of baking soda on hand. I also like to keep a mason jar with a mix of baking soda and 20 to 30 drops of an essential oil on hand for sprinkling whenever I need a little scrubbing action or deodorizing.

5. *Essential oils:* If you're a scent person like me, you associate clean with a scent. If you walk into a room and smell that "clean" smell, it's clean. If you don't smell that smell, it's not clean. Right? Wrong! Hopefully you've figured out by now that this is a lie, but if you still like a scent with your cleaning, embrace essential oils. Look for pure essential oils, not fragrance oils or essential oils with fillers added. A drop or two of lemon and/or peppermint in your vinegar-and-water concoction will elevate your cleaning to the next level, and you'll forget all about that old "clean" scent.

As with anything, there are precautions to take with essential oils. Personally, I don't suggest or recommend ingesting them; they are used only for diffusing and cleaning in our home. Use them with caution around kids and pets. In their pure form, they're extremely concentrated, so I use them heavily diluted and recommend you heavily dilute them too, including in any recipe you find in this book. The general rule of thumb is that for babies, essential oils should not be used. For kids aged two to ten, essential oils need to be diluted. If you have any concerns, purchase the KidSafe essential oils from Plant Therapy.[1] They are made for ages two to ten and are diluted. If you have pets, keep your diffuser away from them and out of their reach (just like you would with a child), and don't diffuse any oils around birds.[2] Talk to your vet if you have any concerns.

On the next page are a couple of my favorite scent combinations for cleaning and diffusing (see page 136 for more ideas). Play around with the ratios and combinations. For cleaning, I typically use 5 to 10 drops in 16 ounces of liquid. For diffusing, it depends on the size of the diffuser, but I usually use about 5 to 10 drops in my diffusers.

6. *Epsom salt:* Epsom salt is a natural detoxifying ingredient. I buy it by the 5-pound bag—Epsoak is the brand I typically grab. If you're a bath lover, add a cup of Epsom salt to a warm bath plus a couple drops of lavender essential oil, soak, and catch up on a book. You'll see what all the fuss is about—the salts draw out toxins, relax muscles, alleviate soreness, and can boost your immunity. If anyone at my house is ill or feeling under the weather, they get an Epsom salt bath and always feel better afterward. I also use Epsom salt to make deodorizing cubes, bath bombs (super fun with the kids and cheap), and Toilet Bowl Bombs (page 123). If you've never tried it, you'll definitely make good use of a bag!

7. *Kosher salt:* I love using kosher salt for cooking whole chickens and seasoning larger cuts of meat, but I sneak a little from that big box for cleaning too. Sprinkle some on your cast-iron pans for an abrasive scrub, and dip a lemon half in it to naturally clean your cutting boards. This is one multipurpose household and kitchen product you need to keep on hand.

LEMON + CLOVE

My absolute favorite scent combination and signature scent. It's homey, warm, and inviting. I use 7 drops lemon and 3 drops clove.

LEMON + PEPPERMINT + LAVENDER

This combo is clean and refreshing. I like it heavy on the lemon and lavender—4 drops each—with just 1 or 2 drops peppermint.

EUCALYPTUS + LAVENDER

If you like the smell of a spa, try this. It's probably the combination they're diffusing. I use equal portions eucalyptus and lavender.

TEA TREE (MELALEUCA) + LEMON + ORANGE

Melaleuca, or tea tree, oil is a natural disinfectant, but it has a strong scent. I like to offset the scent with a little citrus to freshen it up a bit. I use 4 drops tea tree, 3 drops lemon, and 3 drops orange.

LEMON + CYPRESS

I love this combination for washing hardwood floors. The woodsy scent of the cypress and lemon is clean and refreshing. I use 7 drops lemon and 3 drops cypress.

ROSEMARY + CLOVE + ORANGE

If you're looking for the perfect kitchen scent, this is it. The herbal rosemary pairs really well with the clove and orange. I use 4 drops rosemary, 3 drops clove, and 3 drops orange.

CINNAMON + TEA TREE (MELALEUCA)

Cinnamon does a good job of toning down the melaleuca. I use equal parts cinnamon and tea tree for a spicy, clean scent.

8. *Oil:* I like to have olive, coconut, and almond oil in my pantry. If you have tough streaks on stainless steel, put a drop of olive oil on a paper towel or clean cloth and buff the streaks away. Mix olive oil with a little lemon juice for a wood cleaner and polish. I mix almond and coconut oils into my hand soaps and personal care products for soft skin.

9. *Oxygen whitener:* Also known as a bleach alternative, this powder is found in the laundry aisle and works great for whites. Look for a brand that has only one or two ingredients—sodium percarbonate (which is just hydrogen peroxide and salt) is the main one, though it may also include sodium carbonate (a super washing soda). Used in place of bleach and non-chlorine bleach, this powder can *safely* clean laundry, be mixed up in a paste for scrubbing grout, be sprinkled in toilets to whiten, and be used to brighten up dingy carpets. If you're concerned about colorfastness of a fabric or carpet, test the oxygen whitener in an inconspicuous spot first. I recommend my Clean Mama Home Oxygen Whitener.

10. *Rubbing alcohol:* Put a little rubbing alcohol on a cotton pad to wipe down TV remotes and doorknobs. The rubbing alcohol effectively cleans and kills germs. I use it in my granite and marble cleaner and my window and mirror cleaner because it helps dry the surfaces quickly while adding a little cleaning and disinfecting power. Rubbing alcohol can be found in a couple of different strengths—I use the 70 percent concentration and find that it works well.

11. *Vodka:* I know what you're thinking: save the vodka for drinking, not for cleaning! But I've found that the high alcohol content combined with a lack of scent and color makes this an excellent disinfectant. Feel free to substitute rubbing alcohol, but if you have it and can spare it, you'll love it. By all means, grab a jug from a warehouse store and use it to clean and disinfect.

12. *Borax:* Borax is a naturally occurring mineral found where seawater lakes have evaporated. There's some controversy as to its safety, mostly because it can be confused with boric acid, which is not a mineral and is sometimes used as an insecticide. The main concern is due to accidental ingestion, inhalation, and eye contact. As a precaution, take care to avoid inhaling borax in its powder form and keep it away from children. This ingredient can be used in homemade laundry soap, as a laundry booster, and mixed with hot water to get rid of stubborn soap scum. Use caution when mixing it and using it.

Better Household Tools

As you build your detox pantry, you will need some effective and multipurpose tools as well. There's a good chance you have many of these seven tools on hand—this is more about gathering them up and putting them in a place where you can access them easily and have them at the ready, whether that's a caddy or a shelf. I always look for tools that are made from sustainably sourced materials, don't produce waste (like paper towels and cleaning wipes do), and/or can be laundered and reused many times over.

1. *Glass spray bottles:* You'll need these for the DIY recipes I've included later in the book, so keep a couple of them on hand for any cleaning concoction. I love glass spray bottles for a lot of reasons—glass is sustainable (it's 100 percent recyclable), is durable, keeps any cleaning solution intact, avoids the breakdown that occurs with plastic bottles, and just feels good in your hand as you clean. You mean business—you have a glass spray bottle. You might want to look for pump and/or foamer tops for your liquid and hand soaps as well. To clean the bottles, I hand wash them or put them in the top rack of my dishwasher.

2. *Vacuum cleaner (preferably with a HEPA filter and bag system):* This is one tool that I'm a little fussy about, because if you're trying to get toxins out of your home and keep the air that you breathe as healthy as possible, you need a vacuum cleaner that not only removes the dirt but filters out those microscopic toxic particles you can't see. If you're in the market for a new vacuum cleaner, make sure it has some on-board attachments so you can easily switch to using them as you vacuum. I'm partial to the Miele tank vacuum cleaner, though I have the upright as well. The amount of dust and dirt they can store is astonishing, and I love knowing that the HEPA filter keeps the bad stuff contained. No more bagless vacuum cleaners for me.

3. *Dusting wand:* Look for a wand you can reuse. I prefer microfiber or lamb's wool to feather dusters, but choose something that works for you and that you can easily shake clean (outside) mid-dusting and continue using. I love Full Circle's removable-and-washable microfiber dusting wand. It has a wood handle, and the microfiber duster can be tossed in the wash as needed.

4. *Bar mop towels:* These are best for cleaning tasks that you don't want to use microfiber for or if you prefer 100 percent cotton over the polyester blend of microfiber. I use them on kitchen counters daily. They're absorbent, and they wipe up messes effectively.

5. *Flour-sack towels:* These vintage-style dish towels work well for cleaning large surfaces and windows as well as wiping down counters. Thin and wispy cotton, they dry quickly and are lint-free. Keep a stack on hand for spring cleaning!

6. *Microfiber cloths:* For surfaces and windows, these cloths are perfect—no lint, no streaks, just a superb clean. The number one reason I love them? The microscopic fibers pick up more dirt and germs than cotton! Each microfiber cloth has more than three hundred uses, which makes it an ecofriendly choice. Microfiber can be rinsed and wrung out as you're using it, but when it's time to throw it in the wash, you can wash it only with other microfiber cloths. I keep a bucket on top of our washing machine and toss dirty ones in there. You could place a basket or bucket in your laundry room or under a sink if that works better. Then I wash them weekly all together (no fabric softener; just white vinegar) and run a sanitize cycle on the washing machine to make sure I've killed any lingering germs. This keeps the washing machine clean and keeps germs from the cloths transferring to our clothes. Some microfiber cleaning cloths recommend line drying while others recommend drying on low.

7. *Heavy-duty scrub brushes:* If you're scrubbing windowsills or grout, you need a heavy-duty scrub brush or two. I like using wood-handled scrub brushes, and I keep a couple on hand for different types of tasks. Wash them in between uses with a little warm water and soap, and allow them to dry.

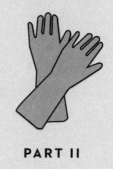

PART II

THE KICK-START WEEKEND DETOX

CHAPTER 6

The Kick-Start Weekend Detox

WE'VE IDENTIFIED THE TOXIC INGREDIENTS LURKING IN YOUR HOME AND WHY THESE pose a risk to the health of your family (and often the planet). We've started to explore some better alternatives for cleaning supplies and learned how to go organic without spending a fortune. I hope you've started to put your Whole Home Detox Pantry together!

Now let's get to work. To make this feel manageable you're going to make a huge impact quickly, with the Kick-Start Weekend Detox. Like a diet detox, it might not feel good at first, but in a day or two you'll see big results. These results will be long lasting too.

I've broken this process down into the easiest format possible, with just three tasks, which I'll walk you through. First, you'll do a quick sweep through your home to get rid of the most harmful products. Second, you'll mix up one quick, easy, and effective DIY cleaner that will help you keep your home clean until you have time to replace every product you've tossed. Third, you'll go through all the products in your home that contain fragrance and toss the offenders.

Follow along at the pace that works for you. You can absolutely take this slowly and replace a cleaner when you run out, but I most definitely suggest going all in from the start. You'll be more likely to follow through with the process if you fully commit, and you'll see results right away rather than slowly, over time.

Ready? Here we go!

GET THE BAD STUFF OUT

Grab a box or a trash bag and take a deep breath (not too deep—your home isn't detoxed yet). Walk through your home and grab each and every cleaning product. I suggest going room by room, starting in the kitchen and moving in the following order:

1. *Kitchen*
   LOOK FOR: dish soaps, dishwasher detergents, hand soaps, and sink scrubs

2. *Bathroom(s)*
   LOOK FOR: disinfectants, mildew removers, toilet bowl cleaners, and shower sprays

3. *Laundry room*
   LOOK FOR: laundry detergents, bleach, spot removers, fabric softeners, and dryer sheets

4. *Utility room/basement/garage*
   LOOK FOR: insect sprays, lawn care products, and drain removal products

5. *Living areas*
   LOOK FOR: furniture sprays and polishes, air fresheners, and glass/window sprays

Move quickly through each room. The key here is not to overthink it! It's easy to dwell on all the money you spent on these products and feel this is wasteful as you prepare to get rid of them. While it's important to be financially conscientious and not wasteful, I think your health and the health of your family are more important. Not to mention, the cleaning system you're going to put into place will save you a lot of money over the long term.

Once you've moved through each room and you've collected these cleaning supplies in one place, take a peek at the label on each product and look for warnings like these:

- Use gloves
- Don't use around children
- Warning, caution, hazardous
- Harmful if swallowed
- Skin and eye irritant
- Do not mix with other cleaning products
- Avoid skin and clothing contact
- Use in a well-ventilated area
- Call poison control if you come in contact with or ingest
- Wear a mask
- Toxic
- Poison
- Flammable, combustible

These are just a few of the many warnings found on common household products. They make it really easy to see what's healthy and what's not. I'm guessing you flipped over a couple of the items in your home already and were shocked to see some of these warnings.

If you see one or more of these warnings on a product, put that product in the box. Don't second-guess this decision—you're making a conscious effort to improve your home and clean it in a whole new way. Don't forget: you'll replace each of these products with a better alternative.

Once you've boxed up the products, put them in your garage or a storage area, and as soon as possible bring them to a household hazardous waste facility or recycling center in your area. Now give yourself a huge pat on the back! Just by removing these products from your home you're already well on your way to better indoor air quality and a less toxic home environment. Even though you might not smell the chemicals in their sealed containers, remember that smell from the aisle at your grocery store? The toxins are releasing themselves into the air even when the bottles and boxes are sealed. If you or a family member has an unknown or undiagnosed sensitivity to chemicals, you or that family member may even feel better within days of removing the products.

Now it's time to arm yourself with a new cleaner to use while you get a whole new system in place. Remember to give yourself an encouraging pep talk—you've just made a huge improvement in your life and in your home. Keep it up!

KICK-START WEEKEND TASK 2

MAKE A REPLACEMENT ALL-PURPOSE CLEANER

My biggest hang-up when I switched to safe cleaning products revolved around illness. I thought, *What if someone pukes? Or gets influenza? How can I clean the house without my disinfectant spray? What happens if there's a germ, or ten million, lurking somewhere? How will I clean properly?*

If you have these same fears, I found that it helped to start with a perspective check. Your home isn't intended to be a completely germ-free environment. Unless you're performing surgeries, common household germs are okay and help to build your immunity. Keep in mind that you just need to keep your home clean, not sterile.

The two options I've included next for a new all-purpose cleaner will reduce germs, especially ones that can cause sickness, like if someone in your house gets the flu or if you have raw chicken out on your counter. Those germs can be taken care of just as effectively with either of these sprays as anything you used before. Mix up either one for any cleaning you need to do over the weekend and into the next week. If you need a little scrubbing power, add a sprinkle of baking soda to the surface after you spray on either of the cleaners and give your surface a scrub. You might even enjoy using these so much that you keep them permanently in your pantry as your clean-just-about-everything products. Later in the book, I'll show you how to make these cleaners in a larger batch that lasts longer.

SIMPLE ALL-PURPOSE VINEGAR-BASED CLEANER

This concoction is perfect for cleaning most surfaces, and it has germ-killing benefits because of the vinegar. Caution: do not use this on marble, granite, or other stone surfaces because vinegar is an acid and can slowly etch the stone. You'll want to use the recipe on page 66 on those surfaces. This is my basic vinegar formula; you'll see it with slight variations throughout the book.

¾ cup water

¾ cup white vinegar

Optional: 10 drops essential oil (lemon and lavender is one of my favorite combinations for masking vinegar; I also like lemon and clove, or just straight lemon)

In a glass spray bottle, add all the ingredients and shake the mixture. Spray it on, and wipe it off with your preferred wiping cloth. (I love using microfiber cloths for bathrooms and dusting, and bar mop towels and/or flour-sack towels in the kitchen.)

SIMPLE ALL-PURPOSE
SOAP-BASED CLEANER

This concoction is perfect for cleaning any surface and is safe to use on stone. This is my basic soap-based cleaner; you'll see it with slight variations throughout the book.

1½ cups water

1 to 2 teaspoons liquid castile soap

Optional: 10 drops of essential oil (if you use a scented castile soap, you can enhance it further with essential oils; citrus scents like lemon, bergamot, and grapefruit are delightful)

In a glass spray bottle, add all the ingredients and shake the mixture. Spray it on, and wipe it off with your preferred wiping cloth (again, I love using microfiber cloths for bathrooms and dusting, and bar mop towels and/or flour-sack towels in the kitchen).

CHECK YOUR FRAGRANCES

As we discussed earlier in the book, it's important to be careful with *any* fragrance. Your final task for the Kick-Start Weekend Detox is to look for hidden fragrances in your home that are *not* in cleaners. Go room to room again, looking for the following items and putting them into the box with your old cleaners:

- Air fresheners
- Plug-ins
- Room sprays
- Candles
- Wax melts
- Perfumes
- Body care products
- Hair care products
- Car fresheners

Looking at each label, box up anything that lists "fragrance" or "parfum," and remove it from your home. We'll take a closer look at your other products later—they're not safe from the chopping block yet.

But for now, you're done! Take a minute to check in with yourself. How do you feel after getting rid of those items? Like I said, it may take a few days to come to terms with the big changes you're making, but if you trust the process, I know that in a few weeks you won't even miss those products!

CHAPTER 7

Five-Minute High-Impact Changes

BEFORE WE GET TO THE FULL ROOM-BY-ROOM DETOX, LET'S TALK ABOUT THE MOST effective way to keep toxins *out* of your home. This one is common sense: don't bring them in! I have ten very simple changes you can make in just five minutes to radically improve the safety and health of your home. Five minutes sounds too simple, doesn't it? That's the thing: by looking at your habits and rituals, you'll see that it doesn't take long to make a change. The flip side is that without making this change, it might affect the rest of your life.

Also, if you skipped ahead in the book and came to this section because you want to put in just a little bit of effort before really going all in, this is your chapter! Start here, and once you see how easy it is to make these changes and you see the difference it makes in your life, I hope you'll continue.

CHANGE 1

TAKE YOUR SHOES OFF AT THE DOOR

Did you know that your shoes track in more than just dirt? Numerous studies have proven this point, but there's one study by Dr. Charles Gerba, microbiologist and professor at the University of Arizona, and The Rockport Company that found on average more than 400,000 units of bacteria on the bottoms of shoes and almost 3,000 units on the insides.[1] The researchers found *E. coli;* meningitis; diarrheal disease; *Klebsiella* pneumonia, a common source for wound and bloodstream infections as well as pneumonia; and *Serratia ficaria.* (Yikes!) When I tell you that the soles of shoes are said to be dirtier than a toilet seat, that alone should encourage you to drop your shoes at the door. The good news is that this dirt is easy to remove—a simple vacuum and/or floor washing will remove the germs from your floors and you can rest assured that you're no longer walking on a toilet seat.

CHANGE 2

WIPE PETS' PAWS WHEN THEY COME INSIDE

We all love our pets, but pets that go outside and come back in potentially track into your home all sorts of dirt, fecal matter, pesticides from parks, and anything else you hope to leave at the door when you remove your shoes. The simplest way to eliminate this isn't to get your pets to wear shoes; simply wipe their feet off at the door. In the winter and spring, when there's a constant stream of mud and muck coming in, this might be a necessity where you live, but keeping the outside stuff outside isn't that difficult and will pay off for you and for your pets. (You don't really want them to lick off that dirt do you?)

I know this sounds like an annoying change to make, but here's a quick and easy way to make this just a little thing you do when the pup comes back inside. Keep a microfiber cloth at the door, dampen it, and wipe off the pet's feet with that. Change the cloth daily or as needed. You can also use the recipe for pet wipes on page 176, and if you don't want to deal with paw-cleaning cloths, use natural baby wipes or paper towels.

WASH YOUR HANDS FREQUENTLY

Hopefully this is something you already do, but it's a good reminder to teach kids to wash their hands frequently throughout the day. This is something I instilled in our kids from a young age. Any time they walk through the back door, they know to take off their shoes and wash their hands. This can be done after playing outside, coming in from the bus, and coming home from shopping, a friend's house, or work. Get your hands wet with warm water, add a little soap, and scrub the palms and backs of your hands and up the wrists. Not only is this the best thing you can do to prevent yourself from getting sick; it's also the best way to keep germs and toxins out of the home by washing them down the drain.

BRING IN SOME PLANTS

Did you know that houseplants are natural air purifiers?[2] This is such a simple way to add a little life to a corner of a room and clean the air at the same time. Start with a plant or two in a living area, and as you find a plant that thrives in your home environment, add another one, continuing until you're officially one of those "plant people." NASA scientists have found that plants can actually absorb toxic chemicals, such as formaldehyde, pesticides, biological pollutants, and radon, to name a few. In the 1960s, Dr. B. C. Wolverton conducted plant studies with NASA and found and rated more than fifty plants that absorb and purify the air.[3]

A few favorites for ease of growing and efficacy are

- Areca palm
- Lady palm
- Rubber plant
- Rhododendron

Pick up a plant the next time you're at your home improvement store. Give it a little love, and it will take care of you!

USE AN AIR PURIFIER

This isn't necessarily a five-minute change, but it's one that can be plugged in in five minutes, and it's such an important aspect of making sure the air in your home is clean. Effective air purifiers clear the air of allergens and dust particles as well as more dangerous substances, like mold, asbestos, off-gassing furniture and paints (VOCs), and other harmful toxins. There are many different types of air purifiers that range in price from less than a hundred dollars to thousands of dollars. We have a whole-house air purifier, and I can tell you that it makes a huge difference in the air quality in our home. One of my favorite features is that I can change how it filters the air. Ours is controlled through the furnace thermostat, and I can adjust it to run 24/7, once every three hours, or once every hour. If someone is sick, I bump it up to 24/7, or if I've dusted or vacuumed, I'll run it continuously for a couple of hours and then put it back to every three hours. It has a HEPA filter so it snags microscopic particles, dust, pet dander, and airborne toxins that make indoor air more polluted than outdoor air. Since we spend up to 90 percent of our time indoors, this can pose a problem.[4]

If you aren't ready to invest in a whole-house system, or maybe you're renting, there are a variety of small and effective air purifiers available. My suggestion is to put one in your bedroom first since we spend so much of our lives sleeping. I like the Dyson, AIR Doctor, and Molekule brands of air purifiers. The Molekule unit is unique, as you can easily move it from room to room, and it has a yearly filter subscription that ensures you'll stay on top of your filter replacements.

If you or someone in your house has asthma, allergies, or other sensitivities, I highly recommend at least a small air purifier for the bedroom. If you aren't ready to get an air purifier quite yet, make sure you change the air filters for your furnace regularly; you'll find that cuts down on household dust along with snagging those minuscule toxic particles.

CHANGE YOUR FURNACE FILTERS REGULARLY

Furnace filters do a good job of removing air particles and dirt, but they only work when they're ready to "accept" that dirt. Some filters require changing monthly, while others require changing quarterly or biannually. Figure out what your schedule is and make a note on your calendar or in your planner so you stay on schedule. Buy a couple of extra filters and keep those filters changed regularly.

FILTER YOUR WATER AND MAKE SURE YOU CHANGE THE FILTERS ON SCHEDULE

This is more of an overall physical health change, but a water filter can remove up to 99.9 percent of contaminants and impurities in your tap water, including lead and chlorine. There are many water filter systems to choose from, and finding out what's in your water is a helpful first step. The EPA requires testing in July for all towns, cities, and municipalities. (If you're on a well, testing is not required.) Choose a filtration system that fits your budget, and make sure you change the filter on schedule so you can take full advantage of its health benefits. Some options are a pitcher or carafe filter, an in-the-refrigerator system, an under-the-kitchen-sink or faucet setup, reverse osmosis, or a whole-home system.

CHANGE 8

VOC stands for *volatile organic compound,* and VOCs are found in paint and a whole bunch of other things we bring into our homes. Basically, you inhale them in the "new" scent of a new car or new furniture, carpet, paint, clothing, etc. We'll talk more about VOCs later, but for a start, make a change with the paint you apply in your home. The next time you paint a room, grab the "Zero VOC" variety instead of the regular or even "Low VOC" paint.

Did you know that conventional paints off-gas for years? And what are they off-gassing? A variety of chemicals that can include xylene, ethyl acetate, formaldehyde, methylene chloride, and more. You can find Zero VOC paint at every paint store and across most brands, so this switch is a snap. You can paint a room during the day and sleep soundly in the room that night—the smell is insignificant in comparison to what you may be used to. You'll find no difference in the quality and performance of the paint, and this little change will take no effort to make. I've been using Zero VOC paint since we moved into our home in 2009, and I can tell you that there's no difference in wear or performance, and I sleep well at night knowing the paint isn't off-gassing.

CHANGE 9

STOP USING PESTICIDES

The most dangerous chemicals in your home or garage? The weed killer, the ant traps, the foggers, the insect sprays—all those chemicals designed to keep the "scary insects" out. I am the first person to throw in a "But what about those wasps and that wasp nest?" or "I can't deal with spiders." I don't care how they're kept out of my home—just get them out! Chemicals keeping our lawns lush and green should also be checked for safety. It's time to throw out all your pest management sprays and solutions.

How can this be a five-minute task? If you didn't already round these up in the Kick-Start Weekend Detox, run around and locate every insect and pest control item and toss it. Do the same for your lawn and weed-control products. If you feel extra motivated, change your lawn service to one that uses natural alternatives (see a few suggestions in the Toxic Ten list, pages 35–36) and/or cut back on treatments.

For bugs, I provide some natural solutions and product recommendations in part IV, but one of the best solutions I've found is a bug zapper. It's large, plugs in, and uses UV light to attract just about every insect imaginable—especially mosquitoes. We have it by our back patio—the zapper, along with citronella candles, which add a nice ambience, keep the bloodsuckers away. Try Aunt Fannie's brand too, which offers all sorts of natural pest control solutions, from a roach spray and insect cards to an all-purpose insect spray, an ant spray, and fly traps. As an added bonus, all of Aunt Fannie's products are rated A by the EWG.

OPEN THE WINDOWS

This is such a simple little thing and it takes two seconds to carry out, but it's one of the best ways to air out your home and recirculate some outside air with the inside air. Homes are more airtight than ever with sealed windows and doors, and we run the air-conditioning or our furnaces year-round. Do you know what might be in your indoor air at any given moment? Radon, mold spores, formaldehyde, VOCs, carbon monoxide, to name a few. Make a point of opening at least one window or door daily to let that fresh air filter into your home. If it's winter, even cracking a window helps. The fresh air will feel good, and it will naturally freshen your house sans air fresheners.

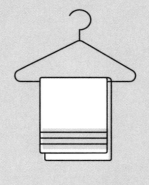

PART III

THE ROOM-BY-ROOM TOTAL HOME DETOX

CHAPTER 8

The Room-by-Room Total Home Detox

AS WE EMBARKED UPON YOUR HOME DETOX, WE STARTED WITH THE MOST IMPORTANT step: getting rid of the cleaning supplies that had toxic chemicals in them. Good riddance! Perhaps you've also started to make some swaps, put a few five-minute changes into effect, or simply are cleaning your surfaces with that lovely all-purpose cleaner you made.

Now it's time to really investigate and question everything in your home. Instead of blanket statements and declarations of what's good and what's bad, I'm going to help you transform your home into a safe environment. I'll show you the facts and make recommendations, then you can choose what works for you now, what will work later, and what you're going to forego completely. This is about picking the changes that are easy and fun for you and giving yourself a break about the rest! The goal here is to build lasting habits, to be mindful about why each change is being made, to give yourself time to test-drive new products and ways of doing things, and to pick what is right for your needs.

And because I can't do anything in my home without making the most of my time and energy, we're going to do a little cleaning and decluttering while we're at it. One of the best parts of this detox (besides just getting the toxins out of your home) is how much *less* you'll have in your home. How's that for an added bonus? Toxins out of the home *and* some sneaky decluttering in the process.

We'll go room by room and at your own pace. Work as quickly or as methodically as you need to. We'll go through each room with a little more care this time to really figure out what you have lurking (or not) behind the cupboards and in the drawers. Each home section will include subsections to guide you through. Here's what you can expect:

WHAT TO LOOK OUT FOR

This will be a quick overview of products you should toss or have already tossed.

SIMPLE SWAPS

Like the swaps in chapter 3, these are tried-and-tested replacements for the toxic or harmful products you've been using. I'll point to my favorite DIY products as well as my favorite store-bought products.

CLEAN AND DECLUTTER

This is a step-by-step process to clean and declutter your spaces.

RECIPES

You'll find DIY recipes at the end of each section if you want to make up some replacement products yourself—try them all or pick and choose! In all honesty, I feel silly calling some of these "recipes."

Consider them cleaning methods and mixes. It's a whole new world out there when it comes to cleaning your home, and please, please, if a recipe says it's for the kitchen but you think it would work well in your bathroom, have at it and mix things up. Find a solution that works for you and go with it—don't let a title hold you back.

QUICK TIPS

These sidebars will give you something you can do *today* to make an area or room safe.

THINK ABOUT IT

The reality is you're probably not going to be able to take care of *everything* immediately. In this section, I'll give you some thoughts on the specific space and what you can do to make it safer—maybe today, maybe when you use up an old product, or maybe down the road.

We'll start with the kitchen and then move through your home methodically to ensure you really, truly detox your home, and declutter in the process. If there's a room or area that doesn't pertain to you, just skip over it and move on to the next section. Think of this part of the book as a safe-home checklist.

One last thing before we get going: I've found it's helpful to have a set of guidelines to follow as I move through a detox. I've put together the Home Detox Guidelines to help as you move forward. When in doubt, refer back to these six statements, and they will point you in the right direction.

I'm so excited for you to see consistent progress and real results. Are you ready?

HOME DETOX GUIDELINES

1. Eliminate any product that has toxic ingredients. Make it your mission to be a supersleuth when it comes to decoding ingredients.

2. Use and consume *less*. Buy things with fewer ingredients, and use products that are multipurpose.

3. If you don't love it or need it, don't keep it.

4. When you make a purchase, buy a quality product that will stand the test of time. Stop buying plastic products—look for natural materials, like glass and wood.

5. Establish daily and weekly routines to keep up with the mess and grime. Doing so will keep your home cleaner longer, and you'll realize that you never needed all those toxic cleaners anyway.

6. Love the home you're in, and make sure it's as safe and comfortable as it can possibly be with what you have today. Don't worry about what you can't afford to change right now—make the changes that you *can* make. And as you're able, make more changes. Remember: this will not happen overnight!

CHAPTER 9

Kitchen

THE KITCHEN IS SUCH AN IMPORTANT PART OF THE HOME. IT'S WHERE WE GO TO GATHER, where we nourish ourselves and our families, but there are also so many potential areas of concern. From the space under your kitchen sink to your food storage containers and pots and pans to the sponges, scrub brushes, powders, soaps, sprays, aerosols, and other cleaners, it can be hot mess of toxins. We'll get rid of any offending items and replace them with better alternatives so that you can feel good about spending so much time in the kitchen.

If you're looking to change how and what you eat too, you can control most of that from your refrigerator, but I'd like to take that a step further and say, "Change what you eat *and* change what you allow into your kitchen." Let's detox your kitchen for both optimal health and lasting change.

What to Look Out For

Let's start by looking at the most harmful products in the kitchen:

- Hand soap
- Dish soap and dishwasher detergent
- Kitchen disinfectant

If you already got rid of these during the Weekend Kick-Start Detox, good job! Perhaps you held back on these because they don't seem that bad—after all, they're meant for use around food and on our hands, right? I remember thinking that way too. But after I learned that these products are commonly full of fragrance and other toxic chemicals, I realized it's safer to just take a hard pass.

If these items are still in your kitchen, take another look at their labels. If something lists "fragrance" as one of the ingredients, get out a trash bag or a box and toss it in. A couple of other common ingredients to look for are phthalates, triclosan, ammonia, and sodium hydroxide. If you see these, you're better off tossing it.

What about products that list essential oils as the fragrance? Are these okay? Look for "pure essential oil" or "organic essential oil" as an ingredient as well as a claim that the company does not use synthetic fragrance.

In the next section are some alternatives for what to use instead. If you don't have time to run to the store to replace products or to make a homemade version, whip up a quick batch of the All-Purpose Vinegar-Based Cleaner (page 65) for your immediate cleaning needs.

Simple Swaps

- *Hand and dish soaps:* Make your own (see pages 99 and 100) or look for a brand that doesn't use any artificial fragrance, is plant based, and doesn't include parabens. EO, Everyone, Rebel Green, and Better Life are brands that are committed to keeping the good stuff in and the bad stuff out.

- *Dishwasher detergent:* Look for one that doesn't have bleach, fragrance, sodium hypochlorite, anti-foaming agents, or phosphates. Unfortunately, there aren't many on the market that don't include these. Even the ones that claim to be ecofriendly really aren't. I've mentioned these two before because they fit the bill for safety and convenience: Seventh Generation Free and Clear Dishwasher Detergent Packs and Grab Green Fragrance-Free Dishwashing Detergent Pods. They are my top choices. You can also make your own (see page 101).

- *Kitchen disinfectant:* Get rid of it now! That old disinfectant has no business being around you or your food. Mix up your own simple, nontoxic all-purpose disinfecting cleaner (see page 95) or try using just hydrogen peroxide with a sprayer top, and use it liberally. Don't want to DIY this? I like Seventh Generation Disinfecting Multi-Surface Cleaner (and it's rated A by the EWG).

- *Scrub brushes and sponges:* Look for products made with natural materials. I especially like plant-based sponges with a scrubby side made of loofah. Wood-handled scrub brushes with heads that can be removed and sanitized in the dishwasher are best. Full Circle brand scrub brushes and Twist brand sponges and sponge cloths are natural, plant-based options.

I recommend running the brush heads and sponges through your dishwasher every evening. It's a super simple nightly task if you have a dishwasher, and it keeps the bacteria off your surfaces.

If you don't have a dishwasher, place your sponge in a dish of water in a microwave for one to two minutes. Allow it to cool, squeeze out any excess water, and let it dry.

- *Paper towels and bar mop towels:* This is going to sound drastic, but I recommend swapping out your paper towels for reusable towels, which will help reduce waste and save you money. I love using bar mop towels on kitchen counters for daily cleaning. If you're not familiar with them, bar mop towels are typically white, superabsorbent terry-cloth towels. Use them with a spray cleaner or dip them in a small bowl filled with warm water and liquid castile soap for a more thorough clean.

  To make using cloth towels as easy as paper towels, place a lidded glass storage container on the counter where a paper towel dispenser would normally be kept. I roll up bar mop towels to easily access them. You could use a small basket or open container with any type of cloth you prefer.

  Put a hook on the inside of the door under your kitchen sink to hang damp cloths while they're drying. When they're dry, put them in a basket or hamper until you have a load of kitchen towels to launder. No more stinky kitchen towels!

  Prefer a sponge? Try sponge cloths, which are made of a thin sponge-like material but are larger than a sponge. (Skoy cloth is an option that can be put in the dishwasher for disinfection.) You can also swap out your traditional sponges for plant-based natural sponges, or do what I do and keep both these options on hand.

Clean and Declutter

Keeping a kitchen clean is important for health safety, but it's also so much more enjoyable to cook and entertain in a space that works efficiently and logically. Follow these simple steps to get your whole kitchen clean and organized once and for all. Use the following checklist as a guide to take you through a complete clean-and-declutter session in your kitchen. I recommend tackling the tasks in this order because it breaks up the kitchen logically so you can handle one or two spaces a day over the course of a week. Or you can lump them all together on a Saturday.

Keep reading for tips and specific instructions for moving through the cleaning and decluttering process.

CHECKLIST

- [ ] COUNTERS, SURFACES, UTENSILS, AND SMALL APPLIANCES
- [ ] OVEN AND SINK
- [ ] REFRIGERATOR AND FREEZER
- [ ] MOST-TOUCHED AREAS
- [ ] PANTRY AND FOOD STORAGE
- [ ] FLOORS
- [ ] UNDER THE KITCHEN SINK
- [ ] ORGANIZATION
- [ ] CABINETS AND DRAWERS
- [ ] STORAGE AND LABELING
- [ ] KITCHEN TOWELS AND CLOTHS
- [ ] PREPARATION AND PRACTICE

Counters, Surfaces, Utensils, and Small Appliances

- First, completely clear your counters. Keep a basket or a bag handy for donations or things to sell later.

- Place small appliances and anything else you have sitting on the counters on your kitchen table. This is the time to edit these items! Remember number three of our guidelines: "If you don't love it or need it, don't keep it." Ask yourself these questions: How often do you really use each of these items? Do you enjoy using them? How old are they, and do they work as well as they should? Could any of these items be stored in a cabinet?

  If you don't use and access the item daily, it probably doesn't belong on the counter. (There may be exceptions—for example, the heavy, awkwardly shaped, and often beautiful KitchenAid mixer.) If you don't use it daily but on a regular basis, store it in a cabinet. If you realize you really don't even find it useful, put it in a bag to be tossed or taken to a thrift store (if it's still in good working condition).

- Do a quick declutter of kitchen utensils. If you have doubles or utensils that aren't in peak condition or utensils you know you haven't used in a while, put them in your donate or sell bin, and toss the ones that are chipped, discolored, or falling apart. If you have plastic utensils, consider upgrading to stainless steel and/or wood.

- Once your counters are clear, mix up a small container of warm, soapy water, take a bar mop cloth or sponge, and wipe them clean.

- Dry as you go and put back just the necessities.

- Now that the counters are clear, decluttered, and clean, rinse out your cloth, refill your small container with warm, soapy water, and quickly wipe the kitchen cabinet and drawer fronts.

Refrigerator and Freezer

- Next up, declutter and clean the fridge and freezer. Start with the fridge. Take everything out, wipe each item clean, and dry the items as you go if necessary.

- Discard any expired food, and make a note of any plastic storage containers you may want to replace with glass when you get a chance. Move quickly, and put everything back in a way that makes sense and is more organized than it was before you started.

- Once you've finished the refrigerator, move on to the freezer. Empty it out, wipe it clean, and dry as you go. Here too make a note of any plastic containers you may want to swap out for glass.

- Discard any old food you won't use. Make a list of what's in the freezer for meals this next week. If you aren't keeping track of what's in your freezer, this is a good time to inventory the items. Use a dry- or wet-erase pen and board to keep an inventory on your freezer door if you have a stand-alone freezer, or keep an inventory/checklist somewhere else in your kitchen if you store all your frozen food in a refrigerator-freezer combo. A little tracking will help you put a stop to the endless stares into the freezer abyss!

- Put everything back in a way that makes sense. Group like products together so it's easy to locate your freezer items. Store together the frozen fruit and veggies. Put all uncooked meat in the same place. Group together the precooked, ready-to-eat meals. You'll be amazed at how much time you'll save by keeping your freezer organized like this (not to mention the reduction in headaches!).

Pantry and Food Storage

- Take everything out of your pantry or food storage area. Wipe each item clean and dry as you go.

- Discard any expired food. If you find any food that hasn't expired but you no longer will be needing it, put it in a bag to donate to your local food pantry. Simplify this space, and keep only what you use regularly. Found a couple of items that inspire dinner? Put them on your menu plan for the next week. Consider limiting your processed-food intake, and look for whole-food items and recipes if this is something that interests you in this healthy living journey.

- Make a note of what items you might want to transfer to glass storage containers. I love using quart-sized glass mason jars in the pantry. One bag of rice, dried beans, or quinoa will typically fit in a quart jar. You can see the contents, and the foods are being safely stored in glass rather than plastic.

- Put everything back in a way that makes sense. For example, group baking supplies together and cooking supplies together. I have a couple of large lazy Susans in the pantry to keep my baking and cooking supplies organized. This creates more space, and it's easy to access these items. Put your cereals on one shelf and snacks on another. Also, anytime I do a thorough pantry declutter I find that the easiest way to put things back is to group them together on the kitchen table or a counter first and then I assess the items and put them back. I've even been known to label shelves with sticky notes so I can see where things will go and if it makes sense before I put them back.

Under the Kitchen Sink

- Completely empty this space and wipe it out. Hopefully you already removed any questionable cleaners, but if not, now is the time to go through them and get them out of this area.

- Consider how you store your cleaning supplies under the sink. I have a large lazy Susan under the kitchen sink too, for soaps and cleaners, and I keep this space minimal. Here's what I have:

  Hydrogen peroxide with a spray top (for disinfecting)

  Rubbing alcohol (to use in the Marble and Granite Cleaning Spray, page 97)

  Nightly Sink Scrub (page 96)

  Fruit and Veggie Clean (by Rebel Green)

  Castile soap

  Bon Ami (the old-fashioned two-ingredient version)

  A small dish for the veggie scrubber

  A kitchen sink scrub brush

  Extra sponges

  Damp cloths hanging to dry before I put them in the wash

- Keep daily-use items next to the sink. I have a small decorative tray by the kitchen sink (you could use a dish or a small cake stand) to hold hand soap, dish soap, and counter spray. We use these daily, so keeping them accessible is important.

Cabinets and Drawers

- If you have the time, you can take everything out of your cabinets and drawers to take stock. Get rid of duplicates and items you haven't used for months or years. Have a waffle iron but only used it once? Consider donating it, or even better, start making Saturday morning waffle morning!

- If going through everything will take more time or energy than you have, that's not a problem. Instead, look for these specific items:

  PLASTIC FOOD STORAGE CONTAINERS: Disposable food storage containers are typically made from plastic, and while the exposure to your food is short-term, cumulative exposure can be extensive. Limiting plastics exposure is especially important for kids and pregnant women. The American Academy of Pediatrics recently released guidelines based on a "growing body of scientific evidence about how certain chemicals may interfere with the body's natural hormones in ways that may affect [children's] long term growth and development."[1] Particularly, the organization recommended that people limit the use of plastic and plastic containers for food. Start by getting rid of your plastic containers and replace them with glass, stainless steel (I love divided lunchboxes for my kids), and/or other materials for transporting food and storing leftovers.

  PLASTIC FOOD WRAP: The next time you run out of plastic wrap, look for a safer alternative. I love using parchment paper for baking, but I do keep an ecofriendly aluminum foil under the parchment paper if I'm making something especially messy. Beeswax food wrap is another good option, as I mentioned previously in the Toxic Ten list (page 40). If You Care is a kitchen paper goods company. I especially like their unbleached coffee filters, waxed-paper sandwich bags, and parchment paper.

PLASTIC SANDWICH BAGS: Like the plastic food storage containers, plastic sandwich bags are another thing I try to avoid. Instead, I use LunchSkins recyclable/sealable paper bags and washable and reusable silicone food storage bags, such as Stasher Bags, which come in fun colors and a variety of sizes.

NONSTICK PANS: The next time you need a new pot or pan, opt for stainless steel, cast iron, and/or safe nonstick options. Many nonstick cookware brands have chemicals in the surfaces and in the chemical process that, when heated or overheated, can transfer into your food. Those chemicals, polytetrafluoroethylene (PTFE), perfluorooctanoic acid (PFOA), polychlorofluorocarbons and fluoropolymers, can be harmful and may even be carcinogenic and toxic at high temperatures.[2] I'd rather not take any chances and just keep all Teflon products out of our home. I really like GreenPan Minerals ceramic for nonstick cookware.

If you don't already have a cast-iron pan, grab one now. They're inexpensive and will last for generations. I use and recommend Lodge brand cast iron. You may have heard that using cast iron actually leaches a small amount of iron into your food when you cook with it, which is true. However, it's such a small amount, and iron is actually considered good for you. Unless your body is one of the rare ones prone to an iron overload, there's no need to worry that it will have a negative effect on you.

REUSABLE GROCERY BAGS: This is a popular choice that I'm glad to see many people already use! Limiting your exposure to plastics and chemicals is important in household products as well as in food products. Put a couple of reusable, washable shopping bags in the back of your vehicle or in your purse, and you'll be making another improvement without much effort. (See a few more recommendations in the Toxic Ten list, page 41.)

KITCHEN TRASH-CAN LINERS: Look for an ecofriendly, compostable brand, like Evolution Bags, Seventh Generation, or If You Care.

Kitchen Towels and Cloths

- Take out all of your kitchen towels and cloths and put them on the table. Go through them. Like we did with kitchen utensils, this is a chance to edit your collection. Are there any that are getting ratty, have a bunch of holes, or are stained beyond recognition? Toss them. Are there any you don't like using (maybe gifts you've felt bad about getting rid of)? Donate these, and if your mother-in-law asks where the towel is, you can blame me.

- Fold your towels and cloths neatly, and put them away in a way that makes sense for your kitchen habits. I like to keep hand towels in one drawer with flour-sack towels. In a separate drawer, I keep bar mop towels and microfiber cleaning cloths. I like also to fold my towels in thirds vertically and then horizontally and store them standing up to maximize the drawer space.

- If you haven't already, consider investing in a couple of sets of bar mop or dish towels to make ecofriendly kitchen cleaning a little easier.

Oven and Sink

- Now move to the oven. If your oven has seen better days, I have a super simple yet effective method for deep-cleaning it. If you have a self-cleaning option on your oven, I'm not opposed to that, but make sure you can open up the windows and run a kitchen fan to clear the fumes from the high heat and whatever it's baking off your oven.

Use my favorite DIY Fume-Free Oven Cleaner (page 104). Mix up the paste with a spoon, then remove the racks from your oven, and apply the paste to the oven walls with a wet sponge. Take care to avoid any seals, holes, and cracks with the mixture. Let the mixture sit for fifteen to thirty minutes and then carefully scrub it with a wet sponge. Using the scrubbing side, rinse, wipe, and repeat until you've removed the paste and the oven is clean.

- Give your sink a good scrub too. Wet it, sprinkle a little baking soda or my Nightly Sink Scrub (page 96) into it, and scrub the surface with a sponge or scrub brush. Add a squirt of dish or liquid castile soap, scrub a little more, and rinse thoroughly. Spray and wipe your faucet, and dry the sink. Baking soda is gentle yet abrasive and can be used for any sink surface.

Most-Touched Areas

- Wipe knobs, doors, and handles. Use a little bit of rubbing alcohol applied to a soft cloth or cotton pad, and give these spots a good disinfecting.
- Clean and wipe your appliance fronts. Use a microfiber cloth with a couple of spritzes of white vinegar right on the cloth—this will work on any surface to get it clean quickly.

Floors

- Because you've done all this work, there's a good chance your floors got a little messy! Sweep or vacuum up the dirt and crumbs, and give your floors a quick mop if necessary (pages 140–142).

Organization

- The key to keeping things organized in the kitchen is to group like items together. Consider using bamboo drawer organizers to keep items corralled and in place. Don't get too caught up in making everything look perfect—this is organization for real life. Make sure you come up with a better solution than what existed before, so you can keep your spaces neat and tidy. Remember that the less stuff you have, the easier it is to organize!

- Do you need to reconsider the layout of your kitchen so that it works as efficiently as possible? This might be the time to move your dishes to a cabinet by your dishwasher so you can stand in one place to put everything away. Are your coffee supplies by your coffeepot? Make those changes now while you're organizing.

- If you have a lot of decluttering to do and/or a lot of drawers and cupboards, consider dividing this process up over a couple of days—do the drawers one day and the cupboards the next day. I've found it's best not to spread the process over too long a period of time (losing momentum is the worst), but also be realistic about how much time it will take, and give yourself plenty of breaks.

Storage and Labeling

- Once you've organized your kitchen, you might need to add some function to how you store things, and make sure you love the way your storage containers look. If you use products that function well and look good, you'll enjoy the space even more.

- It might help to label your drawers or glass storage containers to make locating items easier. Use a permanent paint marker if you like (find them online or at your local craft store—I use the brand Uni-Paint oil-based paint markers) to write on glass, or use a label maker to label items. It will help the space function better, and the labels will also visually unify the space. If you want to remove the marker or change the label at a later time, simply rub it off with rubbing alcohol or lemon essential oil, then wash the surface.

Preparation and Practice

- Plan ahead and stock up on ecofriendly kitchen supplies, like parchment paper, reusable and/or paper lunch bags, bar mop towels, plant-based sponges, and bamboo paper towels. Make the time to choose the best products for your home and family, and place an order for ecofriendly and safe swaps while it's fresh in your mind.

- Watch for a sale on glass storage containers and then make the switch to them.

- As I said before, stop microwaving anything in plastic containers—the plastic might leach into your food. Take ten seconds to put that takeout into a glass container to heat it up. Want to take it a step further? Reheat items on the stove or in the oven when you can. Buy a teapot instead of heating water in the microwave. Heat leftover pizza in the oven instead of the microwave. You'll be eliminating electromagnetic radiation exposure, and you'll find that your food often tastes better heated up that way too.[3]

DIY Recipes for the Kitchen

· ·

ALL-PURPOSE VINEGAR-BASED CLEANER

This will work perfectly on just about any surface you can dream up—except marble, granite, or stone because the acidity can slowly etch the surface of stone. You may notice this is almost the same cleaner I included in chapter 6, but this recipe includes a higher portion of water.

1¼ cups water

½ cup white vinegar

10 drops essential oil, your choice of scent

In a glass spray bottle, add all the ingredients and shake the mixture. Spray it on, and wipe it off with your preferred wiping cloth.

· ·

DISINFECTING CLEANER

Use this anywhere you need to disinfect—your kitchen sink, your non-stone counters, your refrigerator shelves—and spray freely! Remember, a vinegar-based cleaner like this is *not* safe to use on marble, granite, or stone.

1¼ cups water

¼ cup white vinegar

¼ cup vodka or rubbing alcohol (I prefer vodka for its odorless quality—use the cheap stuff)

15 drops essential oils, your choice of scent (I like citrus scents in the kitchen, so I'll usually use 10 drops lemon plus 5 drops either clove or orange)

In a glass spray bottle, add all the ingredients and shake the mixture. Spray it on, and let it sit for 10 minutes before wiping it off with your preferred wiping cloth.

· ·

NIGHTLY SINK SCRUB

This is one of my favorite cleaning recipes and daily rituals. Once the kitchen is clean after dinner, I do a little sink scrub, and it just gives it that perfect reset at the end of the day. I love lemon and clove for their subtle fresh, homey scent, and you can adjust to suit your taste or omit the essential oils altogether. Use it in the bathroom sink too!

2 cups baking soda

20 drops essential oils (I recommend lemon and clove—I usually use 15 drops lemon and 5 drops clove)

1 to 2 squirts castile or plant-based dish soap

In a container with a lid or a shaker top—a mason jar is a perfect container for this—combine the baking soda with the essential oils. Stir and combine them well (remember, do not add the castile or dish soap yet). Put the lid on the jar, and in the evening when your dishes are done and the dishwasher is loaded up, wet the sink and sprinkle this mixture liberally over the sink. Add a squirt or two of the castile or dish soap at this point, and scrub with a sink-safe scrubber (perhaps keep one under your kitchen sink in a mason jar just for sink scrubbing and you'll look forward to this nightly ritual). Rinse the sink thoroughly.

VARIATION: This scrub isn't just for sinks. Use it anywhere you need a little abrasive cleaning action—add water, cleaning concentrate, cleaning spray, or dish soap, and scrub. Use it dry, sprinkled on mattresses or carpets, as a freshener—let it sit to absorb any odors and then vacuum it up.

MARBLE AND GRANITE CLEANING SPRAY

I'm guessing that you can find more than just marble or granite to clean once you try this recipe—it's amazing! Note that the Simple All-Purpose Soap-Based Cleaner I included earlier in the book (page 66) works well with stone surfaces too, but this is definitely one of my favorites. I use it on small appliances and will even spray it on the garden door to clean the glass from muddy puppy nose and paw prints.

1½ cups water

3 tablespoons rubbing alcohol

1 teaspoon castile or plant-based dish soap (if you want your spray to smell like your dish soap, use that)

In a glass spray bottle, add all the ingredients and shake the mixture. Spray it on, and wipe it off with your preferred wiping cloth.

GARBAGE DISPOSAL CLEANER

Use this in your disposal or drain when it gets a little stinky.

¼ cup baking soda

¼ cup lemon juice or white vinegar

In a glass bowl, stir together the baking soda and the lemon juice or vinegar to make a pasty liquid. The liquid will start fizzing—then quickly pour it down the disposal. Let it sit for at least 5 minutes. Run cold water, then turn on the disposal and run it for 30 seconds.

STAINLESS STEEL CLEANER

We love the look of stainless steel until it's time to clean it. This is the simplest, easiest way to wipe off the grime. Alternatively, you can try club soda applied the same way.

White vinegar

Spray white vinegar directly on a microfiber cloth, and wipe the cloth across the stainless steel in the direction of the grain until you've buffed away any fingerprints and smudges.

STAINLESS STEEL POLISH

Once your stainless steel is clean, it might need a little shine. Use olive oil to brighten it up and to remove any mineral deposits near a water dispenser.

Couple of drops of olive oil

Apply a drop or two of the olive oil to either a paper towel or an old, but clean, T-shirt. Wipe in the direction of the stainless steel grain, and buff it to a shine.

SOFTEST HANDS HAND SOAP

Lots of hand and dish washing can lead to dry skin. If you want soft hands that have been cleaned with natural ingredients, try this simple recipe. You'll see that water is optional (depending on the consistency of soap you desire), so if you want a less expensive version, simply add equal parts water and liquid castile soap. Use a smaller dispenser to ensure that the mixture stays fresh.

Liquid castile soap (enough to fill your container three-quarters full)

1 teaspoon almond oil and/or vitamin E oil

4 drops rosemary, 3 drops clove, and 3 drops orange essential oils; or 10 to 20 drops of your favorite combination

Optional: filtered or distilled water

Pour liquid castile soap into your choice of soap dispenser until it's three-quarters full. Add the almond or vitamin E oil and the essential oils. Also add water if you'd like your soap to have a thinner consistency. Then shake the mixture until it's well combined, and wash your hands!

CITRUSY FOAMING HAND SOAP

Soap at the sink is a necessity! Using lemon or other citrus will eliminate garlic and onion smells, and it mixes well with other food-related odors. My favorite thing about foaming hand soap (besides how much my kids love to wash their hands with it) is how inexpensive it is to make, and once you make it, you have what you need to make it on repeat. For this recipe, you'll need a soap dispenser with a foaming pump.

Water

1 to 2 tablespoons liquid castile soap

10 to 20 drops essential oils (I use 10 drops lemon, 5 drops orange, and 5 drops grapefruit)

Add water to the dispenser until it's almost full, then add the castile soap (unscented or scented) and the essential oils. Shake to combine everything, and wash your hands!

DISH SOAP

If you're looking for a DIY dish soap so you know exactly what is inside that bottle, try using a cleaning concentrate product, like Dr. Bronner's Sal Suds, Branch Basics Concentrate, or EO All-Purpose Soap. Each solution has its own formula for dish soap right on the packaging or the company's website—just add water!

Water per recipe

Cleaning concentrate

In a glass soap-pump or spray bottle (depending on how you'd like to deliver soap to your dishes), combine the water and cleaning concentrate as per the brand's recipe instructions. Shake the mixture, and wash up!

NO-RESIDUE DISHWASHER TABLETS

Is there such a thing as a safe dishwasher soap that doesn't leave a powdery residue or food behind? If you're feeling adventurous, try this tablet recipe. It includes the same ingredients you'll find in many natural brands. I've formulated it to work in both hard and soft water, though I can't promise it will work in your home. But I know it's safe! If you have some silicone ice cube trays, they'll work really well for this recipe. The recipe makes about 30 to 32 tablets.

2 cups baking soda

2 cups borax

Optional, for hard water: up to ½ cup Epsom salt or kosher salt

About ½ cup white vinegar (you might not need quite so much)

20 to 30 drops lemon essential oil

In a glass bowl, combine the baking soda, borax, and optional Epsom or kosher salt. Slowly add the vinegar—fizzing is normal—until the mixture is a thick and almost crumbly consistency. Add the essential oils, combining them well.

Push the mixture into ice cube trays, and allow it to dry thoroughly for at least 24 hours—outside in the sun works the best. When the cubes, or tablets, are thoroughly dry (they should be hard but crumbly), remove them from the tray and store them in a glass jar with a secure lid.

Place one in the soap dispenser of your dishwasher. If you notice a powdery substance on your glassware, you might need a rinse aid (simply add white vinegar to the rinse aid compartment and refill when necessary).

LEMON AND THYME
GARBAGE CAN FRESHENER

Everyone's garbage can gets a little stinky from time to time. This solution is simple to mix up and forms into a hard cube that just sits in the bottom of your garbage can, absorbing those odors naturally. If you have some silicone ice cube trays, they'll work really well for this recipe.

2 cups baking soda

1 cup Epsom salt

¼ cup water (you might not need all of this water)

10 drops lemon essential oil

5 drops thyme, rosemary, or lavender essential oil

Optional: 1 teaspoon dried herbs if you want to make this prettier (use the herb you plan to use as an essential oil)

In a glass bowl, stir to combine the baking soda and Epsom salt. Slowly add the water—fizzing is normal—until the mixture is a thick and almost crumbly paste. Add the essential oils and optional dried herbs, combining them well.

Push the mixture into ice cube trays, and allow it to dry thoroughly for at least 24 hours—outside in the sun works the best. When the cubes are thoroughly dry (they should be very hard), remove them from the tray and store them in a glass jar with a secure lid.

Use them as needed in garbage cans or any space that needs a little freshening up. The freshener will absorb and neutralize odors.

REFRIGERATOR AND FREEZER DEODORIZER

Want something a little more attractive than an orange box in the fridge? Keep "that" smell away with this easy alternative.

2 cups baking soda

Pour the baking soda into a mason jar, and screw a shaker top on it. Or cut out a small circle of fabric, place the fabric over the top of the jar, and secure it with a rubber band. Place this in the back of your fridge so the baking soda can absorb any inadvertent odors. Replace the baking soda seasonally. (If your refrigerator or freezer is especially stinky and you don't know the culprit, remove all the contents and wipe it down thoroughly.)

REFRIGERATOR AND FREEZER CLEANER

Am I the only one who is overwhelmed with bringing all the groceries home and then trying to put everything away? Wipe down your refrigerator before you go grocery shopping, and you'll thank yourself when you return and can just slide the goods in with ease. This cleaner is for those times when you need to really do a deep cleaning. Empty the fridge out, put the drawers in the sink to soak, and give it and your freezer a thorough cleaning.

4 cups warm water   **1 teaspoon baking soda**
1 teaspoon liquid castile soap

In a glass bowl, combine all the ingredients. Wipe down the shelves and walls with a well-rung-out microfiber or dish cloth soaked with this cleaning solution. Dry if necessary.

FUME-FREE OVEN CLEANER

This recipe needs a disclaimer because it can get a little messy—follow the directions to a T, and make sure you wipe as you go. I recommend cleaning the glass-door portion of your oven separately.

½ cup warm water

¼ to ½ cup baking soda, enough to make a paste

1 tablespoon liquid castile soap

In a glass bowl, combine all the ingredients with a spoon, adding just enough baking soda to produce a paste. It will expand a bit in volume. Then follow the cleaning instructions on pages 91–92, in the "Oven and Sink" section.

FOOD-SAFE GRILL CLEANER

After every grilling session, heat up the grill and let the food particles burn off. Scrape the racks with a grill brush and let the grill cool. If your grill needs a good deep clean, try this food-safe method.

1 cup warm water

¼ to ½ cup baking soda

White vinegar

In a glass bowl, mix the warm water and baking soda into a paste. Remove the grill racks and apply this mixture to them. Scrub with a scrub brush in a utility sink or outside in a tub.

Soak a cleaning cloth with white vinegar and wipe down the grill. Rinse everything and repeat if necessary. Dry thoroughly.

Quick Tips

Transferring your pantry and cupboard items into glass storage containers will reduce your exposure to plastic as well as make it easier for you to see what you have on hand. It might take some time to get all of your pantry organized in this way, but maybe you have a collection of mason jars left over from a previous canning project or from your wedding. Put them to good use with your rice, oatmeal, and quinoa; your baking soda and sugar; and your cereals.

Think About It

We're working hard to not expose our families to harmful chemicals, and to choose better alternatives. This applies to the food we put in our bodies as well, so it's worth taking a minute to apply what we're learning to our eating habits.

According to Michael Pollan, author of *In Defense of Food: An Eater's Manifesto*, four of the top ten diseases that kill most people (coronary heart disease, diabetes, stroke, and cancer) "can be traced directly to the industrialization of our food."[4] This in and of itself should give us pause and cause us to take a look at what's going on the table and into our stomachs. Sugar is

continued . . .

one concern that many of us watch out for, but other ingredients, like monosodium glutamate (MSG), corn syrup, pesticides, and GMOs, pose concerns for our health too.

If this is something you're already taking into consideration with your eating habits, yay! If you haven't even thought about a whole-food diet—containing "whole," or real, foods that haven't been processed, such as fruits, vegetables, lean meats and fish, brown rice, whole grains, etc.—there are many resources that provide a plethora of tools, recipes, and suggestions. A couple I highly recommend: Lisa Leake's 100 Days of Real Food—I love this website (100Days ofRealFood.com)—as well as her books. Danielle Walker at Against All Grain (AgainstAllGrain.com) has helpful information for anyone dealing with immune-related diseases, but I have found her recipes, cookbooks, and insight work for everyone. I've also had success with Melissa Hartwig's Whole 30 (Whole30.com) for simply resetting taste buds and metabolism. For my family, I've found that the best rule of thumb is to read the ingredients on any box, looking for five or fewer ingredients in any packaged product. This means our family stays away from sodas and sugary drinks; we choose organic produce when possible (a local CSA—community-supported agriculture—or farm is a great way to get seasonal produce); we only use natural sugars, like maple syrup and honey; and I make most of the things we eat from scratch.

This approach to eating might be more time consuming, but it's a change that's better for our health, because the less processed our food is, the healthier we'll be. Even if the only obvious difference is that we feel better, that's enough for me!

CHAPTER 10

Bathroom

'M GOING TO JUST TELL YOU RIGHT NOW THAT I AM NOT A FAN OF CLEANING THE BATH-room. I am, however, a big fan of a *clean* bathroom, so I've devised quite a few ways to clean a bathroom quickly and safely. The bathroom is an important area to master, but it's just as important to make sure you clean it with products that won't make you feel light-headed or give you a headache. Most bathrooms are small and not well ventilated, so spraying a mold-and-mildew concoction can be equated with fogging a home for termites. Don't take any chances! I have plenty of ways you can avoid spreading any germs without needing a hazmat suit!

Bathrooms are a hotbed of germs, mold, and mildew. If you're a person who likes to sanitize everything (like I was), you probably spray surfaces really well and then wipe them up and move on to your next surface. However, that process is flawed when it comes to most cleaning products—the directions state that the solution must stay wet on the surface for ten minutes to disinfect and kill germs. Do you set a timer and check that? I never did. So not only did I fill my lungs with toxic chemicals; I didn't even eradicate those germs I was so anxious to get rid of.

While you're working on your bathroom, it's also important to take a closer look at your personal care products. The last time the United States passed a major law to monitor or regulate ingredient safety in personal care products was 1938. I'll do the math for you: it's been more than eighty years. What's worse is that more than 80,000 chemicals are currently being used in personal care products in the United States.[1] In other words, we are unsure of the safety of thousands of chemicals being used today. Other countries have tested and banned many of these chemicals and ingredients, but the United States hasn't. Don't wait for someone to tell you that an ingredient isn't good for you. Do your own research, keep reading, and when in doubt, throw it out.

Bathroom cleaners and personal care products are some of the worst toxic offenders. Let's get rid of these items. You'll feel better knowing you've eliminated the potential risks, and you'll be able to use safe, simple products for both your bathroom and your body.

What to Look Out For

The most harmful products in your bathroom are:

- Toilet bowl gels
- Sanitizing sprays
- Mold and mildew removers
- Any products with bleach or ammonia in the ingredients
- Most conventional personal care products, including many lotions, shampoos, conditioners, body washes, feminine care products, and perfumes

If you didn't already get rid of these during the Kick-Start Weekend Detox, now is the time! Toss them in the trash and move on. If you're unsure about an item, look on the label for any of the terms we discussed in chapter 2, including "fragrance," "sodium hydroxide," "sodium lauryl sulfate," "sodium laureth sulfate," "formaldehyde," "phthalates," "antibacterial," and any caution symbols or text that say things like KEEP OUT OF REACH OF CHILDREN, WARNING, or USE IN A WELL-VENTILATED AREA. Since most bathrooms don't have adequate ventilation, consider how the very act of cleaning a bathroom could adversely affect your health. Every spritz and spray counts.

Still not sure? If the label doesn't say "plant based" and/or "human safe," it probably isn't. Look up the product on the EWG database or the Think Dirty app.

Sephora recently launched a CLEAN AT SEPHORA seal that indicates which products they sell are made without sodium lauryl sulfate, sodium laureth sulfate, parabens, formaldehyde, formaldehyde-releasing agents, phthalates, mineral oil, retinyl palmitate, oxybenzone, coal tar, hydroquinone, triclosan, or triclocarban. And all skin care, makeup, and hair care items with the CLEAN AT SEPHORA seal contain less than one percent synthetic fragrances.[2]

Again, you are the only one looking out for your home's safety, so protect yourself and your home with what you purchase and use!

Simple Swaps

- *Bathroom cleaning tools:* Use plant-based sponges, natural scrub brushes (made from wood, not plastic), and simple, old-fashioned tools. Our grandmas knew what they were doing so many years ago—elbow grease is one of the best cleaners, especially in the bathroom. I think sometimes we want things clean without having to actually clean them. The cleaner that promises something is clean once it changes color? That cleaner is full of all sorts of nasty ingredients. If it sounds too good to be true, it probably is. Keep with the cleaning ideas I'm providing, and you'll find that it really isn't that difficult after all.

- *Soaps:* Switch out your hand soaps, body washes, and bar soaps. Bonus: castile soap and plant-based soaps have very little or no soap-scum buildup. Do you know what that means? Less scrubbing!

    Like in the kitchen, swap out the hand soap at your sink for something you make yourself (see pages 99, 100, and 124) or look for a brand that is plant based, doesn't use any artificial fragrance, and doesn't include parabens. (See page 44 for product recommendations.)

- *Toilet cleaning discs:* You're going to want to stop using these for a number of different reasons. The first is that if a child or pet gets into the water, they're coming into contact with lots of chemicals, artificial colors, and bleach. That water also makes its way into the environment and contaminates.

    Let's use a better method for our porcelain, shall we? Clean your toilet without really cleaning it by pouring ½ to 1 cup white vinegar in the toilet bowl, let it sit for an hour or so, and give it a little scrub if necessary. Or my favorite? Use a bleach alternative (I like Molly's Suds): put a scoop right in the bowl, let it sit overnight, and give it a good scrub in the morning.

- *Toilet brushes:* Do toilet brushes gross you out? I'm with you. I used disposable wands for years, but I've quit this not-so-green habit. I use a Pumie (a pumice stone on a wand, just for toilets) on hard-water stains. By keeping up with the toilet cleaning weekly I don't find a need for the industrial toilet cleaners.

I also have a small brush inside its storage container beside each toilet, and I use either Earth Friendly Products Toilet Cleaner or just my disinfecting spray (Simplest Bathroom Disinfectant, page 120) and a quick scrub. The secret to clean toilets? Weekly scrubbing and knowing your water situation. If you feel like you get hard-water stains if you clean weekly, clean every other day, or every other day with also a little scrubbing action and a sprinkle of baking soda.

- *Disinfecting sprays:* I've found that hydrogen peroxide is just as effective for disinfection as any of the commercial sprays on the market. Pop a spray nozzle onto the hydrogen peroxide bottle and you're set!

- *Shower curtains:* When it comes time to replace a grungy shower curtain, instead of buying another plastic one, opt for a washable fabric liner. Plastic shower curtains are made of polyvinyl chloride (PVC), which can off-gas for months—just think of that new-plastic smell. Fabric liners are easy to find, generally cost less than twenty dollars, and dry quickly too. Besides the obvious health benefits? You can wash them repeatedly with ease.

- *Plastic bathtub liners:* If you use bathtub liners, look for ones that are PVC-free.

- *Bath mats:* If you have rubberized bath mats, consider solid cotton the next time you purchase them.

Clean and Declutter

Go through everything in your bathroom to determine what to toss and what to keep. I recommend staying in one bathroom and completing it before moving on to the next (if you have more than one bathroom), simply to avoid being interrupted and having all your bathrooms in disarray at 10 p.m.

Here's your bathroom checklist—keep reading for tips and specific instructions for moving through the cleaning and decluttering process.

CHECKLIST

☐ COUNTERS AND SURFACES

☐ FLOORS

☐ CABINETS, DRAWERS, AND MEDICINE CHEST

☐ STORAGE AND LABELING

☐ LIGHT FIXTURES, WINDOW TREATMENTS, BLINDS, AND VENTS

☐ PREPARATION AND PRACTICE

☐ TOWELS

Counters and Surfaces

- Start by completely clearing bathroom counters and surfaces, including bathtub rims and shower shelves. Keep a basket or a bag handy for donations, and the trash for items to toss.

- Edit this space while you're clearing it. For cleaning supplies, if you can't bear throwing away a full bottle of a not-so-ideal cleaner, make a list of new products to replace this with when you've used it up. Look at the other items. Do you have five bottles of half-used lotion? Combine the contents into one or two bottles and recycle the rest. Do you have a bottle of perfume or body wash that someone gave you but you don't like how it smells? Put it in the donation box. You'll feel better once you see the formerly cluttered counter looking so much emptier!

- Spray a cloth with a mirror cleaner (Peppermint Pop Glass and Mirror Cleaner, page 119) and wipe the mirror clean. Same for the medicine cabinet if you have one.

- Mix up a small container of warm water and castile or dish soap, and use it with a small cloth to completely wipe down the counters, especially if they have caked-on hair spray or toothpaste. If you have marble, granite, or other stone surfaces in the bathroom, you can also use my Marble and Granite Cleaning Spray (page 97).

- If the tub or the sink needs a good scrubbing, use my Nightly Sink Scrub (page 96)—it's perfect for both kitchen and bath use.

- Thoroughly spray the toilet with Disinfecting Cleaner (page 95) and wipe it down, from the tank to the floor. Unless you haven't cleaned the bowl lately, there's no need to do so in this particular clean. But if you're like me, with two little boys, staying on top of the toilet can feel like a daily chore. As I mentioned earlier in the book, one of the easiest fixes is to keep a mason jar of oxygen whitener in your bathroom (available at CleanMamaHome.net). Sprinkle it in, let it sit for fifteen to thirty minutes (or even overnight if it's really bad), and scrub it with a brush.

- Spray the shower and bathtub with Simple All-Purpose Vinegar-Based Cleaner (page 65) or Disinfecting Cleaner (page 95) and wipe them down. Again, unless a deep clean is needed, there's no need to do more during this clean.

- If you have time, wash the shower curtains and bath mats.

Cabinets, Drawers, and Medicine Cabinet

This is a biggie. We keep lots of personal care products in our bathroom drawers and cabinets, so I realize this might be a project that will take more than one day. But it's also super important and an area that is often overlooked.

Look at all your personal care products and assess what can stay and what should go.

- If you have time, pull everything out of your bathroom cabinets and drawers. On the counter or the floor, organize them into groups of products:

    Hair care (shampoos, conditioners, mousses, hair sprays, etc.)

    Body and facial care (body washes, face washes, toners, lotions, sunscreens, body scrubs, shaving creams, deodorants, etc.)

    Makeup (foundations, mascaras, eyeliners, blushes, eye shadows, etc.)

    Dental care (toothpastes, floss, mouthwashes, etc.)

    Feminine care products (pads, tampons, cups, etc.)

- Even if you don't have time to go through everything, look at the labels for the following particular ingredients, and this is just to name a few (you'll notice that some of these are the same no-nos as on my cleaning products list):

benzalkonium chloride	fragrance (synthetic)	phthalates
coal tar	hydroquinone	retinyl palmitate
flavor (synthetic)	mineral oil	retinol
formaldehyde (present when other preservatives are listed)	paraben	talc
	petrolatum	toluene
	petroleum	triclosan

The US Food and Drug Administration has guidelines in place, similar to the EPA with cleaning products, but they don't test cosmetics for safety.[3] The EU has banned more than 1,400 chemicals in cosmetic products, while the US has banned only 30 to date.[4] When I learned this, I looked at every product in my drawers and cupboards differently and tossed more products than I'd like to admit.

- Feeling hard-core? Do a clean sweep now and replace the bad stuff with products that are safe for your body and will also make you look and feel great.

> I love Beautycounter for personal care products and makeup you can 100 percent trust. The owner of Beautycounter, Gregg Renfrew, is a mom who, like me, thought everything was safe. When she learned otherwise, she set out to do things differently with Beautycounter. "We're committed to a health and safety standard that goes well beyond what's required by U.S. law: We've prohibited the use of more than 1,500 questionable or harmful chemicals through 'The Never List™'—all while ensuring our products perform and that they're as indulgent as any other luxe shampoo, lipstick, or oil in the market."[5] If you want a quick and easy way to swap out your toiletries and makeup products, this brand is it. I love their lip gloss, makeup, kid products, hair care products, and sunscreen.
>
> I use an electric toothbrush—I find there's less waste and my teeth are cleaner for it. Also, and I know this might be controversial, especially if you work in the dental industry, but fluoride is something I don't buy in dental products. A naturally occurring mineral, fluoride is one of the most toxic substances—less toxic than arsenic but more toxic than lead. It's also in most US tap water, so we get it inadvertently as well.[6] Do your research on whether or not you think fluoride is an additive that you need. I love Schmidt's Naturals toothpaste—I buy the Wondermint for our whole family.

Feminine care products carry a big warning because most of them are bleached. Consider switching to reusable options and/or organic cotton pads and tampons to avoid chemical exposure from fragrance and bleach. Companies like DivaCup, The Honest Company, Lola, and Seventh Generation are some places to start.

- While you have everything out of the drawers and cabinets, do a quick wipe down of both the insides and the exterior surfaces. Use a cotton pad dampened with rubbing alcohol to wipe handles, knobs, doors, and switches and switch plates.

- Put back the products you're keeping in a way that makes sense to you. I like to group like items together in drawer dividers and baskets. Less is more—keep what you know you'll need and simplify the amount of products you use daily. Fewer products means fewer ingredients to worry about. Toss or recycle the products you'll no longer be using.

Light Fixtures, Window Treatments, Blinds, and Vents

- Dust and clean light fixtures.

- Dust and/or launder window treatments and blinds.

- Remove any vents if you can and wash them. If you can't remove them, use a long-handled duster or the wand of your vacuum cleaner to grab the dust and dirt that's built up.

- Dust and clean walls from the ceiling to the floor—I love a long-handled duster for this task.

- Dust and clean any display shelves—put back only what you use and love.

Towels

- Pull out all your bath towels, hand towels, and washcloths. Assess if you need to replace some towels or if you have too many. What kind of shape are they in? For tattered towels, save them as cleaning rags or, as I do, for when the kids are sick to lay down a path to the toilet. You can also donate any tattered ones to animal shelters. Check and see if your local shelter could use a donation.

- Make a note of how many towels and washcloths you need to replace. I recommend four or five per person; this takes into account a daily shower, with each towel reused one time and all towels washed one time a week. If you want to switch to organic cotton towels, now's the time.

Floors

- Vacuum the bathroom floor and vacuum the baseboards. Use your crevice tool to get the corners and edges.

- Wash the baseboards and floors. I will typically do this by hand with a small container of warm water and castile soap because my floor space is small, but you can use your preferred floor-washing method. Wash the baseboards first, rinsing out your cloth under running water several times during the process. Start at the farthest corner from the door and move toward the door.

Storage and Labeling

- Store stocked-up items in baskets or bins to keep everything organized and easy to locate.

- I love using glass apothecary jars in the bathroom for cotton balls and other items used daily. Transferring these items to glass storage is a healthier choice than the plastic containers they often come in, and the jars look pretty too.

- Label the jars or other storage containers when necessary so products return to their home.

Preparation and Practice

- Plan ahead and stock up on toilet paper, tissues, and toiletries. Make the time to choose the best products for your home and family, placing that order for ecofriendly and safe swaps while it's fresh in your mind.

- Consider how your paper products are made and what they're made from. Look for bamboo toilet paper to avoid bleach and possible BPA in the recycled paper (it's in the coating on thermal paper that has been recycled, used for receipts, labels, lottery tickets, etc.). Isn't that the craziest thing? BPA in toilet paper? Just when you think you've looked at every potential harmful substance, you find out there are chemicals in toilet paper and other personal products. Toilet paper is one of those things I know people are very particular about. Rebel Green has a bamboo toilet paper that rivals conventional toilet paper with none of the risk.

- Consider an auto-ship service through Thrive Market, Amazon, or direct from a retailer to make it easy on you and to ensure you don't run out of a product.

- If you use plastic garbage can liners, consider just using the garbage can or looking for an ecofriendly, compostable brand, like Evolution Bags, Seventh Generation, or If You Care.

- The best way to keep your bathroom clutter-free? With toiletries and any items on the counters, practice this rule: if you take it out, put it away. It's good to remind ourselves of this rule as well as to teach it to our kids!

DIY Recipes for the Bathroom

PEPPERMINT POP
GLASS AND MIRROR CLEANER

Looking for clean, streak-free windows and mirrors? This quick-drying spray will do the trick! I promise you'll never go back to the blue stuff after trying this. Use a lint-free cloth with it, like a flour-sack towel or microfiber cloth.

1½ cups water

1½ tablespoons white vinegar

1½ tablespoons rubbing alcohol

3 drops essential oil, your choice of scent (I like peppermint or spearmint for windows—there's something about peppermint and clean windows that is just delightful)

In a glass spray bottle, add all the ingredients and shake the mixture. Spray it liberally on windows. For mirrors, spray it on your cloth and wipe the mirror clean from top to bottom.

CITRUS DAILY SHOWER SPRAY

This cleaner will make any shower or tub easier to clean and keep that soap scum at bay. Hooray! Peppermint essential oil is also a refreshing option for this recipe.

1 cup water

½ cup vodka or white vinegar (if you have marble or granite in the shower, use vodka)

10 drops lemon essential oil

2 drops orange or lime essential oil

In a glass spray bottle, add all the ingredients and shake the mixture. Spray your shower or tub daily after showering. No rinsing is required.

SIMPLEST BATHROOM DISINFECTANT

I know that this seems too easy to believe, but plain old hydrogen peroxide (the stuff in the brown bottle) has been shown to disinfect better than bleach *and* it's non-toxic. Feel free to disinfect your tooth-brush with it or gargle with it if you have a sore throat.

Hydrogen peroxide

Attach to the original bottle of hydrogen peroxide a sprayer, then simply spray any surface that needs disinfection. Let it sit for 10 minutes and then rinse or wipe the surface clean.

Icky grout? Spray hydrogen peroxide on the grout, sprinkle the area with baking soda, and scrub, then rinse clean.

MOLD AND MILDEW REMOVER

Every bathroom gets a little mold or mildew from time to time. I'm not talking about the dangerous stuff. I'm talking about the little bit of mold you might see along a grout or sealant line. Here's a simple solution to get rid of that stuff. For this recipe, tea tree oil is important because its natural antiseptic properties help remove mold and mildew. The best method moving forward? Once you have your shower sparkling clean again, stay on top of it with the Citrus Daily Shower Spray (page 120).

½ cup hydrogen peroxide

1 cup water

20 drops tea tree
(melaleuca) essential oil

In a glass spray bottle (or use the original hydrogen peroxide bottle), combine all the ingredients and shake the mixture. Spray it liberally on mold and mildew, let it sit for 1 to 2 hours, then rinse. Repeat the application if necessary.

If this mixture is ineffective or if you just want to jump to the hard stuff, try spraying straight hydrogen peroxide on the mold and mildew.

LEMON-BRIGHT DISINFECTING CLEANER

Lemon is one of the freshest smells there is, and when you start using natural and safe cleaners, you'll find that lemon is your new favorite scent. This cleaner safely disinfects too, making your bathroom fresh and bright! Though, as I mentioned before, don't use any vinegar-based cleaners on marble, granite, or stone surfaces because the acidity can slowly etch the stone. Also, if you prefer, you can opt instead for the Simple All-Purpose Vinegar-Based or Simple Soap-Based Cleaners included earlier (pages 65 and 66).

1¼ cups water

¼ cup white vinegar

¼ cup vodka or rubbing alcohol (I prefer vodka for its odorless qualities—use the cheap stuff)

15 drops lemon or other essential oil (I like the combination of lemon and peppermint)

In a glass spray bottle, add all the ingredients and shake the mixture. Spray your surface and let it sit 10 minutes before wiping it clean.

MINERAL DEPOSIT REMOVER

You know the mineral deposits that hang out around sinks and faucets? Here's how to get rid of them.

White vinegar (enough to saturate a cloth)

Saturate a clean cloth with the white vinegar and wrap the cloth around the fixture. Let it sit for 15 minutes. Remove the cloth and give it a little scrub. Rinse and repeat if necessary.

TOILET BOWL BOMBS

Need a quick fix for cleaning the toilet? Drop one of these in and let it sizzle away. Give it a scrub or just let it sizzle, then flush. If you have some silicone ice cube trays, they'll work really well for this recipe.

2 cups baking soda

⅓ cup citric acid

2 tablespoons hydrogen peroxide

15 drops lemon essential oil

5 drops peppermint essential oil

In a glass bowl, stir to combine the baking soda and citric acid. Slowly add the hydrogen peroxide—fizzing is normal—until the mixture is a thick and almost crumbly paste. Add the essential oils, combining them well.

Push the mixture into ice cube trays and allow it to dry thoroughly for at least 24 hours—outside in the sun works best. When the cubes, or bombs, are thoroughly dry (they should be very hard), remove them from the tray and store them in a glass jar with a secure lid.

Use one per toilet for a quick clean or an in-between-cleaning freshening up.

DIY Recipes for Personal Care Products

I can't talk about making the bathroom safe without giving you a couple of my favorite recipes for everyday personal care products with ingredients you probably already have in your pantry.

· ·

LEMON AND CLOVE FOAMING HAND SOAP

Dirty hands? Clean and safe ingredients? Yes, please! For this recipe, you'll need a soap dispenser with a foaming pump.

Water

1 to 2 tablespoons liquid castile soap

15 drops lemon essential oil

5 drops clove essential oil (if using this in a child's bathroom, I recommend using all lemon or lemon and orange essential oils)

To your soap dispenser, add enough water to almost fill it. Add the castile soap and the essential oils, screw on the foaming pump, and shake to mix it well. Now wash your hands!

· ·

COCONUT LOTION

This is so simple, but it works! I keep a jar on my bedside stand and use it on my face, hands, and feet at night. I also use it with a cuticle stick as a cuticle cream. Coconut oil has been used for thousands of years and even has been shown to reduce eczema and psoriasis. It also just helps with normal dryness of skin without clogging pores.[7]

Organic coconut oil (I use Dr. Bronner's)

Dip your finger in the jar or use a small tool to apply the oil to your skin.

· ·

ON THE SPOT MOISTURE

Rose hip seed oil is a multipurpose moisturizer for even the oiliest skin, and it can heal scars and acne—quite the one-ingredient wonder. I use it on my face. I also put a couple of drops in my hands and apply it to the ends of my hair to control the flyaways and to make it super soft. The Ordinary and Kate Blanc are brands that offer 100 percent organic cold-pressed oil.

Organic cold-pressed rose hip seed oil

Apply the oil to your skin after washing, using a toner, and applying any serums. Add a drop or two to your hands to work it into your hair as needed.

HAND SANITIZER SPRAY

Prefer a liquid for your hand sanitizing needs? Ditch the chemical versions and try this. Keep it in your purse for a quick spritz. The witch hazel is a natural astringent, and the vitamin E will moisturize. You'll need a 3- to 4-ounce container with a sprayer for this recipe.

2 ounces witch hazel

1 teaspoon vitamin E oil

5 drops tea tree (melaleuca) essential oil

2 drops lemon essential oil

In a small container with a sprayer, combine all the ingredients. Shake the mixture liberally to thoroughly combine everything. Spray it on your hands and let it air dry. Repeat as needed.

HAND SANITIZER GEL

This is my kids' favorite hand sanitizer recipe. It cleans, leaves hands soft, and is safe for the kids to apply themselves. You'll need a small container with a lid for this recipe.

1½ ounces pure aloe vera (not the green stuff)

3 teaspoons rubbing alcohol (or up to 1 teaspoon more for a thinner consistency)

1 teaspoon vitamin E oil

5 drops essential oil, your choice of scent (lemon or orange are my favorites in this recipe and safe for kids)

In a small container, combine all the ingredients, attach the lid, and shake it liberally to mix everything thoroughly. Rub it on your hands and let it air dry. Repeat as needed.

WHIPPED EYE AND MAKEUP REMOVER

This one-ingredient makeup remover is wonderful! This can also be used as a body butter. You'll need a hand or power mixer for this recipe. You'll also need a glass jar to store it. I like the Ball 4-ounce baby-food jars, but you can use a larger jar and more of the coconut oil for a larger batch.

¼ to ½ cup organic coconut oil (I use Dr. Bronner's)

In a mixing bowl, mix the coconut oil until it is the consistency of whipped butter. Transfer the "butter" to your storage jar and seal it.

To use it, apply a small amount to your fingers and use it as you would any makeup remover.

FACIAL TONER/ASTRINGENT

Here are my two favorite one-ingredient toners. Experiment with them to see which works best for you. I like the apple cider vinegar for summer and witch hazel in the winter, but you might find you have totally different results.

For combination/oily skin (and for blemishes too): apple cider vinegar (I recommend using Bragg's organic apple cider vinegar)

For dry/normal skin: witch hazel (I recommend Thayers or Quinn's unscented witch hazel with aloe vera)

Soak a cotton pad with either of these products and wipe the pad over your face and neck after cleansing. These both can be applied multiple times a day.

Keep these products in your bathroom (you can decant them into smaller, cuter bottles if you prefer).

SIMPLE SUGAR SCRUB

If you want just a little scrub to make your hands super soft or to use on your feet, knees, or elbows, this kitchen pantry concoction will do the trick.

⅔ cup organic sugar

⅓ cup almond or olive oil

Optional: 15 drops essential oil, your choice of scent

In a glass bowl, combine all the ingredients well. To use, dampen your body and apply the scrub with your hands, scrubbing away any rough skin. Rinse thoroughly.

The mixture can be stored in a glass jar for up to two weeks.

MASON JAR BABY WIPES

If you're looking for a natural and economical version of baby wipes, this is a way to DIY them. You can also use these as on-the-go hand wipes. If you buy tushy wipes for your family, this might be a replacement too, but they are not flushable. You'll need a mason jar with a lid to prepare and store the wipes. You'll also need a storage bag if you wish to take these on the go and an extra container to store the used cloths between washings.

12 clean soft cloths cut into small (6- to 8-inch) squares, or about 12 sheets of paper towels (non-chlorinated)

2 cups water, preferably distilled

1 tablespoon witch hazel

1 tablespoon unscented (baby) liquid castile soap

1 tablespoon fractionated (liquid) coconut oil or almond oil

1 tablespoon pure aloe vera gel (not the green stuff)

Optional: 2 to 3 drops lemon essential oil (not for babies under two years)

In a quart-size mason jar, place all the cloth squares in a rough stack, or if you're using paper towels, cut them in half and stack them up in a neat pile inside the mason jar.

In a large measuring cup, combine the water, witch hazel, castile soap, coconut or almond oil, aloe vera, and optional essential oil. Stir until everything is well mixed, then pour it over the cloths or paper towels in the jar. Secure the jar's lid and shake the jar, swirling the liquid around so the fabric or towels fully absorb the mixture. Pour off any excess liquid and store the wipes for up to one week.

Quick Tips

Microfiber is your best friend when cleaning your bathroom. It's washable, reusable, and effective for quick and deep cleaning. I think microfiber works best when it's slightly damp. If you don't like using microfiber, look for another washable option. As I mentioned before, bar mop towels, flour-sack towels, and old cut-up T-shirts work well too. Remember, let any cleaning cloth dry before tossing it in a laundry basket to be washed.

I wash my cloths with white vinegar added to the fabric softener dispenser. If they need to be sanitized, I wash them on a sanitize setting and dry them on a low heat setting. Follow the directions on your brand of microfiber cloths for specific drying recommendations. When they're in the dryer, I set the washing machine to a clean setting and let it rip. This ensures my washing machine is just as sanitized afterward as my cleaning cloths.

Think About It

Another thing to consider in the bathroom are the chemicals present in your shower water. I know, I know, this is ridiculous. A shower gets you clean—how in the world is *water* contaminating us?

Skin is our largest organ, so it makes sense that when showering or bathing it absorbs everything we douse it in. The EPA has stated that water from showers also vaporizes into indoor air, which is a double whammy: both skin and lung exposure.[8] Research indicates there is high risk of exposure to chemicals in tap water, specifically chlorine exposure. Simple reactions, like irritated eyes, throat, and skin, are definitely concerns, but there are more dire effects, like lung aggravation and cancer development. An *American Journal of Public Health* article states that chlorine has been linked to increases in certain types of cancer and two-thirds of our exposure to chlorine is just from showering.[9]

Thankfully, there is something you can do. Install a shower filter that filters out chemicals, including chlorine, or install a whole-home water filtration system. While writing this book and doing the research, I made this change myself. We originally had a water softener installed plus a water filter on our refrigerator, so I had assumed we were good. After finding out this information, I had a whole-home filtration system installed and reverse osmosis added to our drinking water sources at the kitchen sink and through the refrigerator. The water tastes even better, and I can tell a difference with my hair, but most importantly, we are no longer exposed to chlorine and chemicals.

CHAPTER 11

Living Areas

FAMILY ROOM, DEN, LIVING ROOM—NO MATTER WHAT YOU CALL IT, IT'S WHERE WE ALL hang out at the end of the day. We want it to be comfy and cozy, neat and tidy, but healthy? I'm guessing it hasn't really crossed your mind. Like the bedroom, we tend to spend a lot of time in these spaces, which makes them crucial to the health of your family. So let's clean and declutter them, and put a couple of new habits in place while we're at it, shall we?

What to Look Out For

Luckily, there aren't too many harmful things in this area. Pay attention to:

- Furniture sprays and polishes
- Dust

If you haven't already, toss any products with harmful chemicals, like that furniture spray and polish. This stuff is full of dangerous chemicals.

All of the fabric in the living room—couches, chairs, drapes, rugs—not to mention all the electronics, makes this area dust city. Dust is a major carrier of allergens and airborne toxins. Frequent dusting and vacuuming is the best defense to keep living areas safe and clean. I'll soon take you through a cleaning and decluttering routine that will take care of the dust bunnies!

Simple Swaps

- *Furniture spray and polish:* There are plenty of safe alternatives out there. I like Better Life's Natural Wood Polish as a spray. I also use beeswax or Daddy Van's Unscented Beeswax Furniture Polish for occasional polishing.
- *Dust cloths:* For dusting, use a barely damp microfiber cloth. If you need a little scent, dampen the cloth plus add a drop of lemon essential oil to it.
- *Storage:* Replace plastic storage containers with wicker or wood options.
- *Furniture:* Forego particleboard furniture (the glue might contain formaldehyde), and go without until you can afford solid wood furniture.

Clean and Declutter

The spaces where you rest and relax can take a beating with daily use. Keeping them clean on a rotation is simple, and it can really ease you into a calmer feeling when you finally do get to sit down and relax at the end of the day.

Here's your living areas checklist—keep reading for tips and specific instructions for moving through the cleaning and decluttering process.

CLEAN MAMA'S GUIDE
TO A HEALTHY HOME

CHECKLIST

☐ SURFACES

☐ FLOORS

☐ LIGHT FIXTURES AND LAMPS

☐ MOST-TOUCHED AREAS

☐ WINDOWS AND WINDOW TREATMENTS

☐ ELECTRONICS

☐ PILLOWS AND BLANKETS

☐ PREPARATION AND PRACTICE

Surfaces

- First, completely clear your surfaces. Keep a basket or a bag handy for donations or things to sell later.

- Time to edit! Go through the items you pulled, and toss or donate anything you don't use or love.

- Recycle or donate any magazines and books you don't use or need.

- Clean and dust all surfaces, wiping down with my Citrus Wood Polish (page 139) or the furniture spray and polish products I mentioned earlier on your nice wood furniture.

- Put things back into place after you've cleaned and dusted, but aim to keep those surfaces clear. Use trays and baskets to contain any items that you need to keep out.

Light Fixtures and Lamps

- Clean and dust all light fixtures, lamps, and shades in living areas. Lint rollers work well for fabric lamps.

- Change lightbulbs to ecofriendly ones. This is something I initially fought. I was going to stockpile the old incandescent lightbulbs so I'd never run out. But when my husband replaced a couple of our high-up lightbulbs and said we wouldn't have to replace them for twenty years, I was intrigued. Then when I saw how effective the light was, I was sold. We've switched out all of our lightbulbs to LEDs, and while it was expensive and something we did slowly, over time, it's cost effective and it saves so much energy, making it a green solution. I love that you can choose what type of light your LED bulbs cast too. I like "daylight" lightbulbs for small rooms that I want to make brighter and whiter, like our powder room and laundry room, and warmer tones of LEDs for larger rooms with windows.

Windows and Window Treatments

- Dust and/or launder window treatments and blinds.

- Wash the windows if necessary (and if you have the time). Try the Peppermint Pop Glass and Mirror Cleaner (page 119) or the Clove and Lemon Glass Cleaner (page 139).

Pillows and Blankets

- If needed, wash the pillows, blankets, and cushions in your living areas. Check the labels, and launder these items seasonally, or as needed, if they're washable.

- If you want to just fluff and freshen them, toss your throw pillows and blankets in the dryer for fifteen minutes.

Floors

- Declutter and clear the floors.

- Thoroughly vacuum, and wash floors if necessary. If possible, move furniture around to really get under and get all your floors clean.

- If your carpets look a little dingy, take some time to give them some love. See my recipe for Carpet Freshening Powder on page 138.

Most-Touched Areas

- As you've done in other areas of the house, use a cotton pad or cloth dampened with rubbing alcohol to wipe handles, knobs, doors, remotes, and phones.

Electronics

- Electronics are dust magnets, they can be difficult to clean and keep clean, and their surfaces can be damaged by cleaning them incorrectly. Turn your electronics off before cleaning.

- Use a cotton pad dampened with rubbing alcohol or an alcohol wipe to disinfect remotes and controllers. If they have pesky crevices, use a cotton swab or toothpick to dislodge any debris.

- Use your vacuum cleaner's soft brush attachment to vacuum behind and under a player component. Wipe components down with a soft, barely damp microfiber cloth.

Preparation and Practice

- Add items to your living areas that encourage family time and relaxation: games, books, more pillows, a plant, a diffuser, a salt lamp, etc.

- This is another room where it's good to remind yourself and others that when we take something out, we put it back.

COMFY COZY SCENTS FOR A HEALTHY HOME

I love using a diffuser to safely freshen up the home. Scent conjures up memories and can ease the senses a bit. Here are a couple of my favorite combinations to give your home a cozy vibe.

Diffuser
Water

Essential oils (try one of the following scent combinations)

Per your diffuser's instructions, add water and your preferred essential oil combination. Turn the diffuser on, sit back, relax, and enjoy your safe scents.

SPA SCENT

2 drops bergamot
2 drops eucalyptus
2 drops lavender

WARM KITCHEN

3 drops lemon
3 drops rosemary
1 drop vanilla

CHRISTMAS POMANDER

3 drops wild orange
3 drops clove

A WALK IN THE WOODS

2 drops cedarwood
2 drops white pine
2 drops clary sage

FALL AT THE FARMHOUSE

2 drops frankincense
2 drops cedarwood
2 drops lemon

CHAI TEA

2 drops cinnamon
2 drops cardamom
2 drops clove

CITRUS GROVE

2 drops bergamot
2 drops lemon
2 drops orange

DIY Recipes for Living Areas

. . . .

CLEAN HOME ROOM SPRAY

The fresh smell of lemon combined with a little spicy clove is perfect for living areas. Feel free to substitute your favorite scents.

½ cup water

¼ cup vodka or rubbing alcohol (I use vodka in this recipe because it's odorless and evaporates quickly)

5 drops essential oils, your choice of scent (I use 3 drops lemon and 2 drops clove)

In a small glass spray bottle, combine all the ingredients and shake well. Squirt 2 to 3 sprays of the mixture in any room that needs a little freshening.

. . . .

CITRUS FABRIC SANITIZER SPRAY

Do you love that fabric freshening spray? It's full of artificial fragrance, but here's a simple and safe swap for you to spray liberally on your fabrics. Get creative and try other combinations of essential oils too! And if you're concerned about using water on your furniture fabrics, test this in an inconspicuous area first.

½ cup water

¼ cup rubbing alcohol

2 drops lemon essential oil

4 drops orange essential oil

In a small fine-mist spray bottle, combine all the ingredients and shake well. Spray this on any water-friendly furniture fabric, letting the fabric dry completely before using that piece of furniture.

. . . .

CARPET CLEANER

My carpet cleaner told me this is the only way we should be cleaning our own carpets. It's safe and effective, and it won't build up in your carpets to collect dirt.

Hot water   **White vinegar**

Depending on the size of your carpet-cleaning tank, mix up equal parts of the hot water and white vinegar. Add the water and vinegar to the tank of your carpet cleaner and clean your carpets as usual.

CARPET FRESHENING POWDER

Are you addicted to that chemical-laden carpet powder? Here's a swap that's both inexpensive and safe. You'll need a mason storage jar for this with a shaker lid, or another type of lid with holes in it.

2 cups baking soda

10 to 15 drops lemon essential oil

5 to 10 drops clove or orange essential oil

In your mason jar, thoroughly mix the baking soda with the essential oils using a table knife or spoon. Secure the shaker top on the jar, and *lightly* sprinkle this over your carpets. Let it sit for 15 to 30 minutes. Vacuum up the powder, and enjoy a safely freshened carpet.

CLOVE AND LEMON GLASS CLEANER

Looking for clean, streak-free windows and mirrors? Look no further.

1½ cups water

1½ tablespoons white vinegar

1½ tablespoons rubbing alcohol

2 drops lemon essential oil

1 drop clove essential oil

In glass spray bottle, combine all the ingredients, shaking well. Spray this liberally on windows or mirrors and wipe clean with a lint-free cloth, such as a flour-sack towel or microfiber cloth, wiping the surface from top to bottom.

CITRUS WOOD POLISH

This is a natural cleaner and polish that will make your wood shine.

¼ cup white vinegar

2 tablespoons fractionated coconut oil or almond oil

5 drops lemon essential oil

5 drops orange essential oil

In a small glass bowl, mix all the ingredients, then dip a microfiber cloth or paper towel into it and wipe your wood surfaces, removing any excess polish as you work. Prefer a spray bottle? Just combine the ingredients in a spray bottle instead.

DIY Recipes for Floors

If you're building a new home or if it's time to replace carpeting or flooring, consider safer alternatives to synthetic-fiber or vinyl products, which release VOCs and sometimes formaldehyde for years. Ceramic tile, hardwood, bamboo, cork, and Marmoleum are better choices for your health.

When cleaning wood floors, a product that contains vinegar is merely my suggestion. Please form your own opinion, and try any combination at your own risk. If you're unsure, test a product in an inconspicuous spot. These recipes are meant only for *sealed* or prefabricated hardwood floors, not waxed or unfinished hardwoods. If you have unfinished, waxed, or bamboo hardwood floors, the best approach is to use a microfiber mop pad barely dampened with water. Always check your floor manufacturer's instructions first.

ALL-PURPOSE FLOOR CLEANER WITH VINEGAR

This old-fashioned combination for washing floors works wonderfully if you want to get up close and personal with your floors. I don't use this every week, but when the floors need a really good cleaning, this works quite well. You can use this mixture on most baseboards too.

1 gallon warm water

½ cup white vinegar

2 to 3 drops essential oil, your choice of scent

In a bucket, mix all the ingredients. Rinse your mop head or cloth frequently, and work in sections, thoroughly wiping areas dry with a clean cloth as you go.

REFILLABLE SPRAY MOP CLEANER WITH VINEGAR

This can be used in a spray bottle too, but refillable spray mops are super convenient and work well for daily touch-ups and regular floor cleaning. Make sure to rinse your microfiber pad frequently to prevent streaking.

16 ounces warm water

3 teaspoons white vinegar

1 or 2 drops essential oil, your choice of scent

Add the water to the mop or spray bottle, then add the vinegar and essential oil. Rinse your mop head or cloth frequently, and work in sections, thoroughly wiping areas dry with a clean cloth as you go.

ALL-PURPOSE FLOOR CLEANER WITHOUT VINEGAR

This works on hardwood floors and contains no vinegar. It's enough for a bucket-and-mop application.

1 gallon warm water

2 to 3 teaspoons castile or plant-based dish soap

2 or 3 drops essential oil, your choice of scent

In a bucket, combine all the ingredients. Rinse your mop head or cloth frequently, and work in sections, thoroughly wiping areas dry with a clean cloth as you go.

REFILLABLE SPRAY MOP CLEANER WITHOUT VINEGAR

This can be used in a spray bottle too, with a cleaning cloth, if you prefer. It works on hardwood floors and contains no vinegar.

16 ounces warm water

1 or 2 drops castile or plant-based dish soap

1 or 2 drops essential oil, your choice of scent

Add the water to the mop or spray bottle, then add the soap and essential oil. Rinse the mop head or cloth frequently, and work in sections, thoroughly wiping areas dry with a clean cloth as you go.

LAMINATE FLOOR CLEANER

If you have laminate flooring, you need a cleaner that dries quickly and without streaking—this is it!

Water

White vinegar

Rubbing alcohol

In a glass spray bottle or refillable spray mop, mix together equal portions of each of the three ingredients. Spray or wipe it on your flooring. This combination dries quickly because of the alcohol, plus it cleans and disinfects.

NATURAL GROUT CLEANER

Grout may be my nemesis, but this simple, natural paste whitens in a hurry!

2 teaspoons cream of tartar   **Lemon juice or water**

In a glass bowl, combine the cream of tartar with enough lemon juice or water to make a paste the consistency of runny toothpaste. Apply it to the grout, and scrub with a stiff-bristled brush. Rinse and wipe the grout dry.

Quick Tips

Add a plant or two to this area to naturally clean the air for you (and look pretty!). Look for one that fits the space and works with the amount of light you have coming in through any windows. As I mention in chapter 7, plants are natural air purifiers. Always keep plants away from kids and pets, as some are toxic if ingested.

Remember that HEPA filter vacuum cleaner I recommended? Use it for cleaning drapery (with a drapery attachment) and furniture as well as floors. Pull it out weekly. Thoroughly vacuuming at least once a week will keep the dust and dirt away and make it easier to breathe in and just plain enjoy your living spaces.

Think About It

If you're planning to make a large furniture purchase in the future, look for a company that doesn't use flame retardants and/or materials with formaldehyde.[1] These products can off-gas for years and contribute to health problems. Plenty of furniture manufacturers keep the toxins out of their products; a quick internet search will turn up a healthy selection.

CHAPTER 12

Bedrooms

A BEDROOM SHOULD BE A PLACE OF REST AND RELAXATION AT THE END OF THE DAY. Unfortunately, there are quite a few potential hazards in our bedrooms, but fortunately, I have some simple, quick fixes.

The first and easiest offender in the bedroom is dust. Dust is made up of skin cells, dirt, pollen, pollutants brought in from outside, pet dander, carpet fluff, and particles from bedding and furniture.[1] Dust is a known contributor to allergies and asthma. It loves to collect in bedding and drapes, and since the bedroom is probably not cleaned as often as the kitchen and bathrooms, it can be an easy place for dust to accumulate. Doing a thorough dusting and vacuuming will clear your home of all sorts of allergens, pollutants, and potential problem causers brought in by us and our pets from the outdoors. Of course, dust is throughout the house, but in my experience, it's the worst in bedrooms.

There are also a couple of hidden dangers in bedrooms, which we'll chat about, and I'll give you some information that should help you make decisions on better purchases when you're ready.

As with the other rooms, let's start with a thorough cleaning and decluttering. Then we'll explore ideas that will make your bedroom a safe haven of rest and relaxation. We do spend a third of our lives in bed, after all!

What to Look Out For

In our fight against dust and allergens, these are the three worst offenders in the bedroom:

- Mattresses
- Pillows (including decorative pillows)
- Stuffed animals

Mattresses and pillows are prone to dust mites, the microscopic relative of the spider. We shed skin cells all the time, but we shed the most in our beds, so a bed is the perfect place for dust mites to congregate to eat old skin cells. So gross, I know, but I bet you're going to put protection on your mattresses and pillows now, aren't you?

Putting a mattress pad on your bed and pillow protectors around your pillows not only shields your mattress and pillows but also keeps dust mites, dust, and allergens away. The next step to protecting your mattresses and pillows is to wash your bedding weekly to keep the little buggers away. If you have kids and they have stuffed animals, toss the stuffed animals in the washing machine with the bedding often to keep them clean and dust-free.

In the next section, I'll provide tips on what to look out for when purchasing mattress pads and pillow protectors as well as what brands to seek out. You'll discover that the prices of the safer alternatives are not that much higher than those of other products, but the benefits far outweigh any cost differences.

Simple Swaps

- *Mattress pad/protector:* This product is constructed like a fitted sheet, going over the top and sides of your mattress. Make sure you choose one that's water-resistant if necessary, doesn't contain flame retardants, and is free of PVC/vinyl, latex (unless it's natural latex from a rubber tree), and phthalates. I like Goodnight Naturals Organic Cotton Mattress Pad.

- *Encasements:* An encasement is a fully zippered product that goes all the way around your mattress. Someone in your family may have allergies or you just want to encase your mattresses and pillows to keep dust and allergens away. An encasement also keeps off-gassing to a minimum if you have a newer mattress that you now realize is probably not the best. (Sorry about that!) You can put the encasement over your mattress pad and then just put the sheets on top of that. I recommend the 100 percent organic cotton encasement from Goodnight Naturals so you aren't exposing yourself or your family to chemicals.

- *Pillows:* Pillows are a place to start when making the move to natural and safe alternatives for your bedroom—they're relatively affordable and are a high-impact change. When shopping for new pillows, look on the packaging for the terms "Certified Organic Cotton," "Greenguard Certified," "GOTS" (Global Organic Textile Standard—95 percent of the pillow is organic and no harmful chemicals are used), or "GOLS" (Global Organic Latex Standard—only organic latex is used). Pillows may also be made from wool or down, which are great distinctions. I like Avocado Green's Pillow and PlushBeds' pillows (wool, organic shredded latex, or cotton-encased down).

- *Pillow covers:* Look for pillow protectors made from 100 percent cotton, preferably organic cotton, that have a zippered closure. The Company Store and CozyPure are a couple of brands that carry a 100 percent organic cotton option.

- *Air purifier:* Filtering the air in your home is a smart idea (it was even one of my "Five-Minute High-Impact Changes," detailed in chapter 7). If you're going to start with just one room, a small air purifier in the main bedroom can clean the air while you sleep. Filtering reduces toxins, like formaldehyde and VOCs, as well as dust and allergens. A whole-home air purifier is another solution, but it's also very expensive. Look for a true HEPA filter purification system with at least three-stage filtration. Clean that air, and get a good night's sleep.

- *Himalayan salt lamp:* Want to add some natural air purification to your bedroom? A Himalayan salt lamp provides an ambient glow, and it's believed to purify the air while attracting dust particles. A small light bulb slowly warms the salt, and the salt attracts particulates to it. You can see it working because you'll find dust on its surface. Starting at around fifteen dollars, a salt lamp is a fun gift idea for a friend—or you just might want to add one to every room!

- *Bedding:* The next time you need new sheets and bedding, opt for 100 percent organic cotton sheets. Why? The cotton will be grown sans pesticides—if there's one fabric product you switch to organic, let it be your bedding. You spend so much time sleeping, you shouldn't be sleeping with pesticides. Switch the bedding out for everyone in your family so you all can sleep in pure, untreated cotton. If you have a baby, don't wait until you need new sheets for them. Make the switch now. Their little bodies absorb more, and they sleep more than children or adults. My favorite brand for bedding is Sol Organics. They carry sheets, down comforters, and pillows that are wonderfully soft and luxurious.

- *Mattress:* A new mattress isn't necessarily a "simple" swap. I know it's a big investment. But it's so important that I want to give you all the information here so when you need a new mattress you can make the best choice possible.

  Look for one that's chemical-free. What? Mattresses have chemicals? Yep, they come complete with VOCs (that new-mattress smell), flame retardants, phthalates, and perfluorinated compounds (PFCs)—like those found in stain treatments.[2] All of these things I'm sure are included with the best of intentions, but they're toxins, and since we sleep on our mattresses nightly, over time we absorb those chemicals into our bodies. The chemicals also break down over time and turn into dust particles that move through our homes.

  If you have kids, start with their mattresses. I wish I'd done this research when we were buying crib mattresses; I would have made completely different choices. Organic mattresses will go a long way toward protecting your young children from toxins.

  Look for a mattress made without fire retardants, which are added because the polyurethane foam typically used in mattresses is highly flammable. But the ingredients in the retardants are toxic. With plenty of non-treated mattress options available, it's not worth the risk. Wool has natural flame resistance, so you'll see mattress options with that as well. Like with pillows, a place to start when shopping for a mattress is with these certifications: Greenguard (products with this meet rigorous standards when it comes to emissions from any chemicals, such as VOCs, formaldehyde, and fire retardants); GOTS (ensures a mattress was made with at least 95 percent organic materials and no harmful chemicals); and GOLS (on latex products, ensures only organic latex was used).

  Some brands to start with are Avocado Green, Naturepedic, Tuft & Needle, Goodnight Naturals, and Essentia. If your budget doesn't allow for a new mattress, consider an organic natural latex or wool mattress pad/topper and organic sheets for right now. Remember, just because a company says something is "organic" or "natural" doesn't mean that it is. It needs to be "certified organic" and carry a legitimate seal. It might be made with 100 percent organic cotton, but if the whole mattress contains only 5 percent cotton, that little bit isn't going to benefit you the way you think it will. If you have any questions, always contact the company directly and ask for details.

Clean and Declutter

Go through everything in your bedrooms to determine what to toss and what to keep. I recommend staying in one bedroom and completing it before moving on to the next.

Here's your bedrooms checklist—keep reading for tips and specific instructions for moving through the cleaning and decluttering process.

CHECKLIST

☐ SURFACES

☐ ORGANIZATION

☐ PILLOWS, BLANKETS, AND BEDDING

☐ PREPARATION AND PRACTICE

Surfaces

- Start by quickly clearing the surfaces in your bedroom and picking up anything on the floor that doesn't belong there (hello, socks). Set these items aside to organize later, and keep a basket or a bag handy for donations or things to sell.

- Dust and clean all light fixtures, lamps, and shades. As I mentioned before, a lint roller works really well on fabric shades. Dusting the lamps and shades ensures that the dust falls on the surfaces you'll be cleaning next.

- Dust and/or clean all other surfaces. I like using a barely damp microfiber cloth and a microfiber dusting wand for this task. Dusting always comes first, then we can vacuum up those dust particles.

- Thoroughly vacuum and/or wash floors, including the baseboards while you're at it. If you can move the bed and vacuum under it, take that extra step. If you can't move it, get your vacuum cleaner under the bed as far as you can.

- Open a window while you're working to allow dust to escape and naturally freshen up the room. Again, if it's winter, even a tiny crack will help.

Pillows, Blankets, and Bedding

- Launder pillows, blankets, and bedding if necessary. At the least, toss your bedding in the dryer to fluff it up for fifteen minutes. It will clear some of the dust and allergens, and the heat will kill some germs.

- Put clean sheets and pillowcases on the bed, plus a clean quilt or duvet cover. Save time by getting rid of the top sheet and using a duvet cover with a comforter—it makes bed-making a breeze!

Organization

- Go through the pile of items you picked up earlier. Put any stray dirty clothes into the hamper. Now it's time to edit! If there's something you don't use or love, put it in your donate basket.

- Put away the items you decided to keep.

- If you have a load of laundry waiting to be folded, take care of that now too.

Preparation and Practice

I've found it helps to give myself a couple of rules to keep the bedroom spaces clutter-free. Here are my rules—use any that are helpful to you:

- *Make your bed every single day.* This little step sets the tone for the day, and if you don't accomplish anything else, hey, you made your bed!

- *Don't store laundry baskets with clean (or dirty) clothes in the bedroom.* Bedrooms can be a dumping ground for clothing—both clean and dirty. If you want to feel calm when you step into your bedroom, a pile of clothes doesn't help. Store your dirty clothes in a bedroom closet or in the laundry area in a basket or hamper. Try to fold and put away clothes as you wash them. This will keep your bedroom tidy and keep that overwhelmed feeling of "All the laundry!" away.

- *Use a basket or bowl for must-have items.* Corral jewelry, books, lotions and potions, and other regularly needed items into cute dishes or baskets so the items stay in one spot and look cute at the same time.

- *Clear the top of your dresser, and put a storage system in place to keep it clean and uncluttered.* Keep that dresser cleaned off. If you have a hodgepodge of stuff, use a dish or jewelry box for your jewelry and a tray for your essential oil roll-ons.

HOW TO WASH YOUR PILLOWS AT HOME

Remove all pillowcases and pillow protectors. These can be washed with your pillows, but you'll want to remove them first. Put at least two pillows in the washing machine together to balance the machine and guarantee a thorough cleaning. Use some of the Simplest Laundry Soap (page 165) and set your washer at its largest capacity and on a gentle, warm-water cycle. After the wash cycle is complete, run the rinse cycle again. This ensures all the soap is removed from the pillows. Run the spin cycle again too to remove any excess water, which helps the pillows dry a little more quickly.

If your pillows are foam, you will want to line dry them, because a trip through the dryer would cause the material to melt. Otherwise, toss the pillows into your dryer with a couple of wool dryer balls, which will agitate and return the fibers to their natural state. For other synthetic materials (besides foam), choose a low to medium setting—avoid high heat. Down and natural materials can't stand much heat either, so set your dryer on an air or a low setting, and allow the pillows to dry thoroughly. Stop the dryer every thirty minutes or so to rotate the pillows to make sure they dry evenly.

- *Keep your bedside tables clear too.* Beyond something like an organizing jewelry dish, make sure your bedside tables are cleaned off too. Replace that phone and charger with a book that's on your to-read list.

- *Put a donate basket in your bedroom closet.* Ever try on a shirt that no longer fits or you don't love anymore? Instead of hanging it back up, put it in your donate basket. When the basket is full, donate its contents.

- *Put things away daily.* Maintenance is key to a tidy bedroom. Pick up in the morning after you've made your bed and do a quick tidy in the evening before you jump into bed. It'll probably take less than a minute, and you'll feel fantastic when you walk into the room and it's still clean!

I love using a duvet or comforter on our beds. One of the best parts is being able to launder them at home in lieu of bringing them to a dry cleaner, and a home wash is the safest option for care and maintenance of this investment. There may be a couple of situations in which you'll need to launder a duvet, but for the most part, if you have a cover on it, you can easily freshen up your duvet before you need to all-out wash it.

To freshen up your duvet or comforter, simply put it in the dryer (with or without its cover) on a low heat setting with three wool dryer balls; this will help agitate and return the fibers to their natural state. Tumble the bedding for thirty to forty minutes, stopping the dryer every ten minutes or so to redistribute it. If you want to kill germs without washing the duvet or comforter, put the dryer on a high heat setting for thirty minutes and keep an eye on it, rotating the bedding every five to ten minutes.

To wash a duvet or comforter, first remove its cover (if you use one). Use some of the Simplest Laundry Soap (page 165) and set your washer on a delicate or gentle cold-water setting and at its largest capacity. A front-load washer with a large capacity works the best. (If you have to cram your comforter in and it's a super-tight fit, you might want to take it to a laundromat instead.) After washing it, run it through the rinse cycle again. This ensures all the detergent is removed. I typically run the spin cycle an extra time as well to remove excess water, which helps the comforter or duvet dry a little more quickly.

After the wash and extra rinse and spin cycles, place it in the dryer with some wool dryer balls. If your comforter or duvet is made from synthetic materials, dry it on a low or medium heat setting—avoid high heat. Down and natural materials can't stand much heat either, so set your dryer on an air or a low setting, and allow the bedding to dry thoroughly. Stop the dryer every thirty minutes or so to rotate the bedding to make sure it dries thoroughly and evenly.

DIY Recipes for the Bedroom

. . . .

LAVENDER DRAWER SACHETS

Reminiscent of the sachets your grandma used, these are made with lavender, which will freshen your drawers and keep that musty smell away. Dry your own lavender by hanging stems of it upside down in a dry place, like a closet. Find some small cotton drawstring bags for storage, from an apothecary supply store such as the online supplier BulkApothecary.com.

Dried lavender stems

After the stems have fully dried, place them in a paper bag and shake the dried flowers off the tops. You may need your hands to help with this process. Transfer the flowers into small drawstring cloth bags. Use them anywhere to impart some freshness.

. . . .

LAVENDER AND CEDARWOOD PILLOW AND BEDDING SPRAY

Use this gentle spray to softly scent your pillows and bedding. Spritz lightly while making the bed and when you climb in at the end of a long day. The scent will calm you. Remember, take care when using essential oils around children and in their rooms and play spaces. All of my recipes with essential oils are best used around children aged two and over. Keep these products out of the reach of both children and pets.

½ cup water

¼ cup rubbing alcohol

6 drops lavender essential oil

2 drops cedarwood essential oil

In a small fine-mist glass spray bottle, combine all the ingredients and shake to mix everything well. Spray this on bedding and linens to ensure a good night's sleep.

. . . .

LAVENDER AND EUCALYPTUS
ROOM FRESHENER SPRAY

I love this combination for bedrooms because it's relaxing and it smells like a spa. Feel free to substitute your favorite scents—you'll see another version in the Clean Home Room Spray (page 137).

½ cup water

¼ cup vodka or rubbing alcohol (I use vodka in this recipe because it's odorless and evaporates quickly)

3 drops lavender essential oil

2 drops eucalyptus essential oil

In a small glass spray bottle, combine all the ingredients and shake well. Squirt 2 to 3 sprays of the mixture in any room that needs a little freshening.

CITRUS AND TEA TREE
FABRIC SANITIZER SPRAY

If you need to sanitize or freshen a pillow or a pair of shoes, this spray will become a new favorite. If you're concerned about applying water to any fabric, test this in an inconspicuous area first.

½ cup water

¼ cup rubbing alcohol

2 drops citrus essential oil (lemon, orange, grapefruit, etc.)

4 drops tea tree (melaleuca) essential oil

In a small fine-mist glass spray bottle, combine all the ingredients and shake well. Spray the mixture on shoes and fabrics to freshen, and let the items dry completely.

EUCALYPTUS AND PEPPERMINT MATTRESS FRESHENER

If you're freshening up the bedroom or trying to eliminate the scent of something on your mattress, use this. Vacuuming a mattress seasonally is a good idea to eliminate allergens and dust. If you want to make a little more and store it, simply increase the amounts and store it in a sealed glass jar. Lavender essential oil works well in this recipe too if you prefer it. Also note that you will need a fine-mesh sieve or sifter for sprinkling.

¼ cup baking soda

3 drops eucalyptus essential oil

2 drops peppermint essential oil

In a small glass bowl, stir together the baking soda and essential oils. Using a fine-mesh sieve or sifter, *lightly* sprinkle the mixture over your mattress. Let it sit for at least thirty minutes, then vacuum up the powder using an upholstery or hose attachment on your vacuum cleaner. Clean the attachment both before and after you use it.

Quick Tips

If you don't have a carbon monoxide detector in your home or on the same floor as your bedrooms, pick one up, put a battery in it, and plug it in (having a battery provides a backup in case the power goes out). This is a cheap solution to protect yourself and your family from a potentially deadly gas. The carbon monoxide detector will trace any level of gas, and you can sleep easy.

Think About It

Let's talk for a minute about cell phones. (Here's where I might lose some of you, but stick with me.) Cell phones can be great, and they've become integral to our lives in many ways, but they also emit radio frequency waves from their electromagnetic fields (EMFs).[3] While EMFs have been around forever, information is starting to come to light regarding the dangers of our exposure to EMFs, particularly surrounding cell phones, computers, Wi-Fi, and other electronic devices. My recommendation is to protect yourself and your family while we wait and see what the long-term effects are.

Some experts recommend putting devices in airplane mode at night to keep the electromagnetic exposure to a minimum. I think the safest idea is to keep them out of our bedrooms altogether. I know many people use their cell phone as an alarm clock, but it's safer to use an actual alarm clock. If you need to have it in your bedroom to get a call, don't place it by your bed or your head—put it across the room. At my house, we still have a landline and use that for 90 percent of our phone calls. We also have a charging station for our cell phones in the kitchen.

It's smart to keep other devices, like laptops and Wi-Fi routers, in a room far away from your bedrooms to limit your electromagnetic exposure. We've decided to use a Wi-Fi Kill Switch from Tech Wellness to turn off multiple devices at once. Finally, purchasing an RF shield to block the radio frequency waves is a good idea for laptops and other devices. SafeSleeve is my favorite brand for aesthetics as well as blocking technology, and DefenderShield is another option.

CLEAN MAMA'S GUIDE
TO A HEALTHY HOME

CHAPTER 13

Laundry

DOES ANYONE LOVE DOING LAUNDRY? I USED TO ENJOY IT WHEN IT WAS JUST ME AND my husband, but three kids later with multiple wardrobe changes (sports, workouts, spills, and plenty of other things), it's definitely not my favorite thing. But it's on my daily priority list. Yep, I do laundry each and every day, and what I remind myself while I'm grumbling in my head is that that one load of laundry every day is much easier than the potential baskets upon baskets it would be if I saved it for a week.

You already know that laundry products are pretty much near the top of the toxic list. If you associate clean laundry with a certain scent or product, I encourage you to be open-minded and willing to experiment with some safe alternatives. I too love a basket of clean, fresh-smelling clothes, and we should be able to find a new scent that works well for you. What I'm *not* okay with is clothes that still smell sweaty or appear dirty or dingy just because I'm using a safe option. You will not find that here. There are plenty of safe alternatives, and they smell better too!

Let's get started with what to look for and get rid of, and then move to how you can clean and declutter your laundry room.

What to Look Out For

The most harmful products in your laundry room are:

- Conventional laundry detergent
- Bleach (sodium hydrochloride)
- Fabric softener and dryer sheets
- Stain remover (in liquid or stick form)

You got rid of all these toxic chemicals already, right? If you haven't, toss these products now. As I've said before, many of them have dangerous ingredients, like fragrance and sulfuric acid, which is known to be a carcinogen.[1] Trust me, you'll feel so much better once you have the safer alternatives to use in their place.

Simple Swaps

- *Laundry detergent:* Make your own (Simplest Laundry Soap, page 165) or use the following brand alternatives: Clean Mama Home, Molly's Suds (they make the powder that we use in the Clean Mama Home detergent), Rebel Green, and Better Life.
- *Bleach:* Use oxygen bleach, a bleach alternative. This powder is found in the laundry aisle. Look for one that has only one or two ingredients—sodium percarbonate is the main one, but it may also have sodium carbonate. I recommend our Clean Mama Home product but also Molly's Suds Oxygen Whitener.
- *Fabric softener and dryer sheets:* Choose one of the alternative fabric softeners I list in the recipes (Vinegar Fabric Softener, page 166, or Wet Fabric Softener Sheets, page 167). Your laundry will smell fresh and not one

bit like a jar of pickles—trust me! My favorite for the dryer? Wool dryer balls. Place a few drops of essential oil on them to lightly scent clothes as they dry, plus they reduce static (see page 169). Try some Mini Flannel Dryer Sheets too (page 169).

- *Stain remover:* You'd be surprised by how well liquid laundry soap works on stains. You can also use a bar of castile soap as a stain stick stand-in (see Laundry Stain Bar, page 170).

Clean and Declutter

If you have a dedicated laundry area, chances are you aren't in the habit of cleaning it on a regular basis. Take a little time to organize it and give it a deep clean, and I bet you'll be more inclined to enjoy the washing and folding process. Okay, maybe that's an exaggeration, but at least you won't be putting your basket on top of a sticky detergent ring on your washer.

Here's your laundry checklist—keep reading for tips and specific instructions for moving through the cleaning and decluttering process.

CHECKLIST

☐ SURFACES ☐ PREPARATION AND PRACTICE

☐ ORGANIZATION, STORAGE, AND LABELING

Surfaces

- First, if you have any piles or baskets of clean laundry that need to be folded and put away, do that now. If you have baskets full of dirty clothes, move those out of the way for the moment.

- Clear your laundry area of unnecessary items, and remove everything from the shelves and drawers. Keep a basket or a bag handy for donations or things to sell later.

- As we've done in previous rooms, take time to edit. If you find you have many more hangers than you'll ever use or one too many baskets, toss and donate these and any other excess items you no longer need or want.

- Take stock of what is and isn't working. Need to move something around or need a new container for your safe laundry powder? Make a list and take care of the problem now, while it's fresh on your mind.

- Spray and wipe down shelves and drawers with an all-purpose cleaner (page 65 or page 66) or just a damp cloth, and wipe them dry. Put items back into place.

- Clean your washer and dryer. Wipe the surfaces clean and wipe out the interior as well with a damp microfiber cloth. See my instructions for how to thoroughly clean and sanitize your washing machine naturally on page 168. Vacuum under and around your washer and dryer too, or as much as you're able to.

Organization, Storage, and Labeling

- Group like items together and organize your laundry room to make it work for you.

- Store powders in glass containers and add a scoop utensil to each container. Transfer liquids like vinegar into bottles with a pump or sprayer for easy use. Select pretty containers to make your supplies more attractive, and label anything that needs it. If your laundry products look pretty, you'll be more likely to use them and enjoy them.

Preparation and Practice

- Put the rule we discussed earlier into practice in this space too: if you take it out, put it away.

- Do a load of laundry every day to keep the task manageable. If you have less laundry, or you're spending money at a laundromat and find it gets expensive, do laundry a couple of times a week instead, or just enjoy the fact that you can do multiple loads of laundry at once when most people can do only one load at a time.

- Think ahead and prepare the DIY laundry recipes beforehand so you're ready to go the next time you want to do a load of laundry. Plan a day for putting these products together. Even better, plan a DIY party where you gather some of your friends and make the products together! You'll be spreading the healthy home love and having fun!

HOW TO PLAN A HEALTHY HOME DIY PARTY

Have you ever had a meal-prep party where you gather friends together, make a bunch of soups or casseroles, and then send everyone home with meals that will freeze and last awhile? You could host a similar party for home care products! One of the best ways to encourage healthy home choices is to share your findings with your friends and family. Getting others excited to make changes is easy when you show them how simple and economical it is to make your own home care products, and everyone goes home with a few different options. Fun!

Here's all you need to do:

- Invite your friends.
- Plan a couple of recipes to prepare—my favorites for a party are my Nightly Sink Scrub (page 96) and my Peppermint Pop Glass and Mirror Cleaner (page 119).
- Gather supplies.
- Have a party!

Set up the supplies, complete with the ingredients, bowls, spray bottles, jars, measuring cups, spoons, funnels, and labels. Set up stations for easy assembly and mixing, and have fun! If you plan to make a product with an essential oil, have a handful of options and some guidelines for scent combos (like the suggestions I provide for diffusers on page 136), and let your friends mix and match as they like.

Once you have a couple of friends on board with these changes in their home care, plan regular refill parties, where everyone brings back their bottles and together you refill them and try out other recipes.

DIY Recipes for the Laundry Room

. . . .

SIMPLEST LAUNDRY SOAP

Clean clothes with a product you can make yourself? Hooray! This recipe yields up to 96 loads of clean laundry.

1 bar castile soap, any scent you like, finely grated (I use a food processor)

2 cups borax

2 cups Arm & Hammer Super Washing Soda (sodium carbonate— find this item in the laundry aisle)

1 cup baking soda (sodium bicarbonate)

30 drops essential oils (lemon and lavender, or lemon and clove, are my favorites for laundry)

In a large container, such as a bucket, combine all the ingredients well, taking care to keep the dust to a minimum. Carefully transfer the laundry soap into a gallon storage container. I use a glass container with a lid so it has form and function.

To use, measure 1 tablespoon per load for high-efficiency machines and 2 tablespoons per load for regular machines.

To whiten a load, add 1 to 2 tablespoons store-bought oxygen bleach powder as well (that's the safe stuff).

. . . .

LAUNDRY SCENT BOOSTER

If you love commercial scent boosters, this recipe is for you! It adds scent as well as softens.

1 to 2 cups Epsom salt (depending on how much you want to make)

20 to 30 drops essential oils, your choice of scent

In a glass bowl or a mason jar, combine the Epsom salt and essential oil, stirring to mix thoroughly. Use 1 tablespoon of this in each washer load and wash as usual.

VINEGAR FABRIC SOFTENER

If you love your fabric softener and dryer sheets and love that scent associated with clean laundry, you probably don't want to make the switch to something unscented, even if it's natural. I'm right there with you. I want my laundry to smell clean and fresh. Yet white vinegar does this without any fragrance. Your laundry will smell fresh and not one bit like a jar of pickles—I promise! But you can add essential oils if you truly miss a particular scent.

White vinegar

Optional: up to 10 drops essential oils per 16 ounces vinegar, or 40 drops per gallon, your choice of scent

Add ¼ cup white vinegar to the fabric softener dispenser for each load of laundry. I love this for sheets and towels—it will make your towels unexpectedly soft and fluffy. Plus, it keeps your washing machine fresh.

If you'd like to add essential oils, decant the vinegar into a 16-ounce bottle or gallon jug, with a pump for easy dispensing if you like, then add the oils of your choice, and shake well.

WET FABRIC SOFTENER SHEETS

Prefer a wet fabric softener sheet you add to the dryer? Try using white vinegar in the dryer instead of in the washing machine. You'll need a mason jar with a lid for this recipe.

¼ cup white vinegar

10 drops essential oil, your choice of scent (citrus options work well for this)

20 or so small pieces flannel or cotton cloth (3- to 4-inch squares or rectangles; you can also purchase precut cloths—I like the cloth wipes from MarleysMonsters.com)

In a mason jar, combine the white vinegar and essential oils, shaking to mix them well. Add the cloths to the container, and secure the jar's lid. The "sheets" should absorb the liquid completely. If there's any residual liquid, pour it off into a sink and scrub the sink clean.

Each sheet can be reused a couple of times. Once a sheet is dry from the dryer, just put it back in the jar and it should reabsorb a little liquid. When a sheet no longer becomes even barely damp, that's when to wash it and start over.

All washing machines need to be cleaned weekly or at least once a month. The result is an odorless machine that you know is sanitary. I clean my washing machine after I launder my cleaning cloths to wash away the icky, germy stuff.

Some machines have a self-cleaning option or a separate cleaning cycle. If you don't have these as an option, select the hottest water setting possible. Add ¾ to 1 cup white vinegar to the bleach dispenser of your machine, or fill it to its maximum level. Then select an extra rinse option if your washer has that choice, or make sure to repeat the rinse cycle later. This will ensure that the vinegar will be completely rinsed from the machine.

Once the washing machine has completed its cycle and an extra rinse, wipe out the bleach and fabric softener dispensers. These can be easily cleaned in warm, soapy water in a sink, or you can wipe them down without removing them from the machine using a cloth dampened with white vinegar. Rinse and dry them thoroughly before reinserting them.

If you have a front loader, wipe down the rubber seal on the door, as it is a perfect hiding spot for mold and mildew. Pull back the rubber gasket and carefully wipe down the area with white vinegar and a soft cleaning cloth. Rinse it with a cloth dampened with water and wipe it dry thoroughly with another clean cloth to prevent any moisture buildup.

If you have a top loader, wipe down the inside of the lid and the seal.

Next, wipe down the exterior and control panel of your machine with an all-purpose cleaning spray (Simple All-Purpose Soap-Based Cleaner, page 66, or Simple All-Purpose Vinegar-Based Cleaner, page 65) to remove any dust and dirt buildup. Be sure to leave the door or lid of your machine open to prevent moisture or mildew from forming inside in between loads, and to avoid unwanted smells.

WOOL DRYER BALLS

Wool is naturally antibacterial, making it awesome for use in the laundry. Wool dryer balls reduce static in a dryer and lightly scent your laundry if you add essential oils. The ones I sell at Clean Mama Home are ethically sourced and wonderfully durable. Most wool dryer balls will last 1,000 uses, making them an inexpensive, ecofriendly dryer-sheet alternative.

3 wool dryer balls

6 to 9 drops essential oil, your choice of scent (I use

a deodorizing blend from Plant Therapy or Purify Cleansing Blend from doTERRA)

On each of your wool balls, add 2 to 3 drops essential oil. Let them dry. You also may use the wool balls in your dryer without any scent added if you prefer.

Add all 3 wool balls to a single dryer load.

MINI FLANNEL DRYER SHEETS

If you *need* to use a dryer sheet, here is your safe alternative. It adds a subtle scent to your laundry. You'll need a mason jar with a lid for this recipe.

20 or so small pieces flannel or cotton cloth (2- to 3-inch squares; you can also purchase precut cloths—try MarleysMonsters.com)

20 to 30 drops essential oil, your choice of scent

In a mason jar, stack the cloths, adding a drop or two of essential oil to each one. Keep the lid off the jar until the "sheets" have completely dried—at least a day or two.

Use one or two sheets for each dryer cycle.

Reuse them with renewed oil as often as you like.

LAUNDRY STAIN BAR

I love this easy, natural, nontoxic alternative to stain sticks and sprays. I use it on kids' clothes and dirty pant knees. Try it the next time you have a stain that needs some attention. This solution works best on basic clothing stains that are fresh and not yet set in. You'll need a small soft-bristled scrub brush for this.

1 bar castile (any size) or   **Water**
other plant-based soap

Push the bar of soap up a bit out of its wrapper. Wet the top of the bar under running water or in a dish of water—I like to use a dish because it's more controlled. Rub the wet bar into the fabric stain, rewetting and reapplying as needed. Scrub the area with the small scrub brush if necessary. Launder the item of clothing as usual.

Store the soap bar in the wrapper when not in use; it will dry completely in a couple of minutes after using it.

If you use a liquid soap, not a bar, rub the soap directly into the stain, possibly without additional water.

Quick Tips

Too much static with natural products? Put a safety pin in your wool dryer balls, which will cut the "charge," eliminating static. Also, don't overdry your laundry. When laundry is overdried, it tends to incur static.

Put a drying rack in your laundry room for items that need to be line dried. I have a teeny tiny laundry room with a wall-mounted laundry rack that folds up. It's cute and functional.

Use your laundry detergent as your pretreater too. If you use liquid soap, simply apply it to a stain. If you use a powdered detergent, wet the stain with cool water and sprinkle the stain with your detergent. Stains on white fabrics? Wet the fabric and sprinkle it with oxygen whitener. With all of these treatments, let the mixture sit from thirty minutes to overnight to break down the stain, then launder the item as usual.

Think About It

When you're shopping, look for quality clothing, bedding, towels, and other items that are intended to last.

If you have plastic hangers and are planning to upgrade, look for a more sustainable product. Wood or cloth-covered hangers last a long time and look nicer.

Looking to upgrade your washer and/or dryer? I love having a sanitize cycle on my washer. It makes using washable cleaning tools simple, and it's reassuring to know the items are sanitized and safe to be used again. Another feature I love is the "clean washer" cycle that uses just steam! Make sure the cycle options that are important to you are included on any washer and/or dryer you're considering purchasing.

CHAPTER 14

Entryway/Mudroom

ANY TYPE OF ENTRYWAY OR MUDROOM IS A GIFT IN A HOME. IF YOU HAVE ONE OR both, utilize every nook and cranny of them to make the entry and exit of your home simple yet hardworking. At its most basic, this is where you take off shoes and hang up coats. Everything else is extra, but most important, and regardless of the size, this area should provide a comfortable spot to come in, take off your shoes, and stay awhile.

What to Look Out For

Thankfully, there aren't many harmful things we keep in this area of the house. The things to be most careful of we've already discussed:

- Dirty shoes
- Pets bringing in dirt from outside

As we talked about in the "Five-Minute High-Impact Changes" in chapter 7, shoes carry into your home all sorts of germs, toxins, and pesticides. Dogs coming and going through your door bring in the same. Here are some ideas to help minimize the transport of these unwanted items into your house.

Simple Swaps

- *Shoe mat:* Here's where the shoes will sit. Make sure you have a doormat that functions well and can be easily vacuumed and cleaned. I like washable rugs for high-traffic areas—we have washable wool-blend rugs in the mudroom, at the back door, and in the kitchen. I can't tell you how many times they've been vacuumed and laundered, but they still look like new and they were inexpensive. I have a large decorative rug in the entryway because only guests come in that door. A rug signals to take your shoes off. If you don't have one, make it your goal to get one for this space. If you want to make your guests feel especially comfortable, add a basket with fresh socks or slippers for them to slip on upon arrival.
- *Pet wipes for paws:* Create pet wipes from old cloths or T-shirts (see page 176). Change the cloth daily or as needed. If you don't want to deal with making and washing wipes, you can use natural baby wipes or paper towels.

Clean and Declutter

The entryway and mudroom get daily use, yet this area doesn't get cleaned and decluttered as often as it should. Let's give it some attention.

Here's your entryway/mudroom checklist—keep reading for tips and specific instructions for moving through the cleaning and decluttering process.

Coats, Shoes, and Overall Clutter

- Start by picking up shoes and outerwear: coats, hats, gloves, scarves. Completely empty the coat closet, bench, etc. If any other miscellaneous things are scattered around, pick these up too. Keep a basket or a bag handy for donations or things to sell later.

- Time again to edit! As with other rooms, go through the items. Are there any old shoes or boots your kids have outgrown or that have holes? Any mittens missing a mate? Old coats to get rid of? It's time to toss or donate.

- What is and isn't working? If something isn't working, put a new system in place. Add storage if you need to, and make sure you have a place to hang guests' coats.

- Sweep or vacuum outside the entry area.

- Clean and wipe down any shelves.

- Wash and vacuum the floor.

Organization and Storage

- Group like items together for easy access and attractive storage.
- My biggest issue in the mudroom is shoes—they always seem to collect and pile up! Use baskets or a tray to contain shoes, and keep them to a minimum.

Preparation and Practice

- Put a vacuumable, washable rug in the mudroom. Quickly running over the rug when you vacuum and being able to toss it in the washing machine is key to keeping those outside toxins out.
- If you have a sink in the mudroom, put a safe hand soap at the sink.

DIY Recipe for the Entryway/Mudroom

. . . .

PET WIPES

- Cut up old cloths or T-shirts and store a stack of them in a bucket or basket by the door with a spray bottle of a simple soap-and-water mixture. Alternatively, use a microfiber cloth, dampening it with just water.
- With the moistened cloth, wipe the pet's paws off at the door.
- Reuse the cloth for a day, then put it in a bucket in the laundry area to wash when you have a bucketful.

. . . .

Quick Tips

Keep a lint roller, sweater shaver, and any garment care items in a basket for any clothing mishaps. The entryway or a mudroom is a good place to store these items for easy access.

Think About It

If you have a garage entryway, you may want to put a bristly rug, like coir (from the husk of a coconut) or jute, in that space to wipe shoes on before entering the home. This will keep the icky stuff in the garage.

If you live in a climate where shoe storage would be possible in your garage, don't be afraid to put a shoe rack there. This will keep your entryway or mud-room clear and keep the shoes out of the house entirely.

CHAPTER 15

Garage and/or Basement

THE GARAGE AND BASEMENT ARE TWO AREAS OF THE HOME I'M NOT A BIG FAN OF cleaning, but occasionally they need it. Hiding in these areas are most likely the more toxic cleaners and pesticides, so we'll take a peek at those and turn your basement and/or garage into safe places too.

What to Look Out For

A number of toxic products may be lurking. The most important ones to look for are:

- Pesticides and insect repellants
- Chemical cleaners
- Cans of paints and varnishes with VOCs
- Vehicle air fresheners

All of these need to be properly disposed of. Check your city's hazardous waste options. Old paints you need or wish to hang on to can be decanted into smaller glass jars so they take up less space if you prefer.

Simple Swaps

- *Pesticides and insect repellants:* You already know to rid yourself of pesticides. Aunt Fannie's brand insect repellent is a better alternative (see my Toxic Ten list on page 35 for more information on bug control). To make your own, see my Simple Insect Deterrent recipe on page 182.
- *Paints and varnishes:* Use "Zero VOC" products instead, as you know!
- *Vehicle air fresheners:* If your car is stinky, put a drop of essential oil on a cotton ball and tuck it under your car seat to naturally freshen this space.

Clean and Declutter

If you hate cleaning these seldom used and/or seldom cleaned spaces as much as I do, this is most likely a neglected space.

Here's your garage and/or basement checklist—keep reading for tips and specific instructions for moving through the cleaning and decluttering process.

CHECKLIST

☐ FLOORS AND SURFACES ☐ ORGANIZATION

☐ MOST-TOUCHED AREAS ☐ PREPARATION AND PRACTICE

Floors and Surfaces

- Clear the floor and any surfaces. Keep a bag or box handy for things to donate or sell.

- It's time to edit once more. Lose anything you don't use or love. If you have boxes and bins to go through—split that task up in a way that makes sense for your schedule. If you want to tackle it over a weekend or over a week or two, divide up the boxes and bins accordingly. Less is more: now is the time to get rid of that bin you haven't touched since you moved five years ago. If anything is just taking up space, let it go.

- Vacuum and clean all surfaces.

- Vacuum and/or wash the basement and/or garage floor.

Most-Touched Areas

- Use a little bit of rubbing alcohol on a soft cloth or cotton pad to wipe handles, knobs, doors, and switches and switch plates to give these spots a good disinfecting.

Organization

- Put any systems in place that will help this space. Need bike hooks? Put those in. Would a shelf or shelving system help? Get that installed.

- Group like items with like items, keep only what you need and use, and make sure the clutter is gone.

CLEAN MAMA'S GUIDE
TO A HEALTHY HOME

Preparation and Practice

- Make it a habit to empty the car of anything that you added to it with each return to the garage.

- As I mentioned in the previous chapter, put a rug in the garage for wiping shoes off to keep those toxins out of your house.

- As I also mentioned in the previous chapter, consider putting a shoe rack or shelf in your garage to store shoes and boots to keep your entryway or mudroom clear and keep the shoes out of the house.

DIY Recipes for the Garage and/or Basement

. . . .

HEAVY-DUTY FLOOR CLEANER

This can be used in basements and garages, on both tile and linoleum. Use it when you need a little cleaning boost. You'll love the results.

1 gallon hot water	¼ cup borax (make sure you don't inhale it, and keep it away from children!)
10 drops essential oils, your choice of scent	

In a mop bucket, combine all the ingredients, stirring to dissolve the borax, and mix everything well. Mop the floors as you normally do. Rinsing is usually not required.

. . . .

SIMPLE INSECT DETERRENT

Pesticides are harmful, but insects can be too. Insects don't like white vinegar, and it's safe to use in your home—hooray!

White vinegar

If you have a sudden ant invasion, pour white vinegar into a spray bottle and spray vinegar at the entry points, letting it dry. If you have a little ant-marching session, spray the ants with vinegar and wipe them up, also spraying the exterior and interior points of entry. The vinegar will deter the insects and keep them out of your home.

CLEAN MAMA'S GUIDE
TO A HEALTHY HOME

Quick Tips

Investing in a large shop vacuum might be a good option for cleaning up these spaces. It will contain the dirt and make cleaning a little easier.

While vehicles technically aren't part of these spaces, they do move in and out of the garage (if you can fit them in). As I said earlier, keep your vehicles clean by doing a quick sweep each and every time you come home. Try not to eat in the car to keep the mess to a minimum. If you tend to eat in the car, store a bag in the car to dispose of any trash.

Think About It

While these spaces aren't necessarily used as frequently as other areas in the home, they still need a good cleaning and decluttering. Make this something you do seasonally or at least at the end of summer and at the end of winter. Frequent maintenance makes it easier to function in any space.

Do you have pets? Think about changing to ecofriendly and biodegradable waste bags for your pup, like Poop Bags and bioDOGradable bags, and safe cat litter, like Cedarific Soft Cat Litter (wood based) and Eco-Shell's Naturally Fresh (walnut-shell based).

CHAPTER 16

Daily Habits and Routines for Homekeeping

NOW THAT YOU'VE TAKEN AWAY THE TOXIC CHEMICALS IN YOUR HOME, IT'S TIME TO layer back in a beneficial ritual—a routine. This chapter could go anywhere in this book, but I want you to consider it like a capstone, topping all that you've accomplished so far. Hopefully you're feeling lighter, more free, and empowered by the positive changes you've made. Now we'll make sure those changes stick by putting a cleaning routine in place.

If you follow me online, you know that my simple daily and weekly routines are the foundation of the brand. I'm not the only one who finds calm when the house is in decent order and things are where they should be. I live with my husband, three children, and our dog, so this isn't all about me, but we have some basic routines that somehow help us keep our stuff together and truly enjoy life. Many times it feels like we're just constantly putting out fires—you know the ones: the dishes, the messes, the piles, the laundry. Along with being a haven, your home is in need of constant maintenance, and the people who live in your home (yourself included) are mess makers. You know what? That's *okay!* Embrace the fingerprints, the spills, and the messes, but have a daily plan, and you'll be much less bothered by them.

Daily Habits

Proactive home care is much more effective than reactive home care. It's about what you and your family do daily to make things run more smoothly. Cleaning and picking up is what will keep the mess at a minimum. Your home will be easier to maintain and you'll spend less time cleaning—trust me on this. Through my own experience and through the countless emails and feedback I receive from readers and followers, I've found that it's the consistent effort and a little habit building that keeps a home clean most of the time. If you're familiar with my books and my website, you know that my main advice has always been: every day, a little something. Clean something, but not everything, every day. That little bit of effort will pay off every single day, and it will pay off the most when something unexpected happens, because then you aren't starting with a mess when more piles on top.

A quick story to illustrate what I mean: Have you ever been working on a project or a task and completely in the throes of it only to be sidelined by something unexpected? A simple phone call may turn what you were doing into something meaningless in an instant. A job loss, illness, a death, or maybe it's just a kid coming home sick from school.

For me, it was a Friday morning, when I was relaxing and catching up on some social media work on my computer and had Netflix on in the background. I happened to look up and saw water on the ceiling above me. I took a moment to think about where that water was coming from only to realize that it must be coming from the laundry room. Sprinting up to the laundry room, I saw the puddle of water under the washing machine and started calling service companies to find that no one could service it until the following Tuesday. This could have thrown me off, but since I was caught up on the laundry with the load that was clean in the leaking washing machine, I made the appointment, dried the clothes, and relaxed.

Still, my fear was that with a broken washing machine, it was likely that one of the kids would get the stomach flu. (Am I the only one who thinks like this?) Luckily, the kids remained healthy, but unluckily, the dog broke out of her kennel and was sick in every room throughout the house that had carpet. (Of course the hard-surface floors were spared—ha!)

The next two days were spent with wall washing and carpet cleaning on repeat, and my regular cleaning routine wasn't enforced whatsoever. I was on high alert, sick-dog mode. After the washing machine was repaired, things started to get back to normal. I washed a couple of loads of laundry and started back in on my Tuesday routine of dusting. By Wednesday, everything was pretty much back to normal and things started to click again. The house wasn't in complete disarray because I had been taking care of things the week before.

I've seen this system work for me and for countless others I've worked with. I want it to work for you too. The daily and weekly tasks listed next take just minutes a day, and with a little effort, you'll soon find that they are quite possibly home and life changing.

Here's the schedule for the daily and weekly tasks and how I typically tackle them. Try it out for a couple of weeks, and see how it is to finally feel in control of the mess!

CLEAN MAMA'S GUIDE
TO A HEALTHY HOME

Daily Tasks

Make the Beds

Quickly pull up your bedding and fluff those pillows as soon as you can in the morning. This will help your mind-set for the day. I prefer to forego the top sheet and just use a bottom sheet and a washable duvet cover or quilt. This is especially helpful for little ones when they're old enough to make their own beds. Even if you don't see your bed again until it's time to climb back in it, you'll appreciate that the bed you finally get to crawl into is made.

Check the Floors

Sweep or vacuum as needed, but try to check the floors at least daily. In my house, it seems like the broom comes out after every meal, but it's a quick sweep under the kitchen table and it's put away. If the day is a busy one, I might wait until after dinner and just drag out the broom once. If you have pets, you might need to grab that vacuum cleaner or broom a little more often, especially if it's shedding season, or maybe your furry friend is helpful with picking up the remnants of meals. This is a great small job for kids to take on—teach them how to operate a broom and dustpan and/or a small vacuum cleaner.

Wipe the Counters

Wipe down your kitchen counters after meals and at least once daily, after dinner. I include emptying and loading the dishwasher with this task. Check the bathroom counters to make sure they're clean and cleared off daily. If you keep makeup and beauty supplies out, consider putting them in a basket, or in a drawer instead, to keep the counters clear and easy to clean. A quick walk through the bathroom(s) in your home with a cleaning cloth and an all-purpose cleaner works. This makes it easier to maintain a clean home, and it discourages keeping the counters cluttered in the meantime.

Declutter

Learning to deal with clutter is the number one daily task in our house. I like to avoid feeling overwhelmed by a pile of papers on the kitchen counter or a pile of shoes at the door. Adopt a mantra that works for your home when it comes to clutter. Some good ones are: "Touch it once," "Never leave a room without putting something away," "Sort mail daily," "Put clothes away daily," and "Everything has a place."

Do the Laundry

I'm easily overwhelmed by laundry. As I said before, the best way I've found to address this is to do one load every day, from start to folded and put away. Simplify your laundry routine by using just the basics we've discussed in this book. My must-haves for fresh, clean clothes are laundry powder, white vinegar (for softener), and wool dryer balls to help the clothes dry quickly and to eliminate static.

Weekly Tasks

Monday: Bathroom Cleaning Day

Every Monday I clean bathrooms. I don't wash the floors because I wash them on Thursdays. I find this really cuts down on bathroom cleaning time.

I keep cleaning supplies in each bathroom; you might prefer to tote a cleaning bucket or caddy from bathroom to bathroom. You'll need these supplies for a well-stocked bathroom caddy:

- Disinfecting Cleaner (page 95)

- Peppermint Pop Glass and Mirror Cleaner (page 119)

- Toilet Bowl Bombs (page 123) and a brush—oxygen bleach powder also works really well as a toilet scrub

- Microfiber window cloth

- 3 or more microfiber cleaning cloths for *each* bathroom (1 for counters, 1 for tub/shower, 1 for toilet)

Follow this quick method for speed cleaning your bathrooms:

1. Clean the mirror.

2. Thoroughly spray the sink, toilet, and tub/shower.

3. Move on to the next bathroom, and repeat these first three steps until you've sprayed each bathroom.

4. Go back to the first bathroom, and wipe each surface and scrub the toilet. Repeat in each subsequent bathroom.

Tuesday: Dusting Day

I do my best to only keep out things that we love and need. Especially with little kids, I have a minimal amount of "stuff" on display just so I don't have to worry about anything happening to items. Having uncluttered surfaces makes dusting so much easier. And dusting weekly makes it simple to keep on top of it.

My preference for dusting is using microfiber cloths and a dusting mitt (which you can find in the Clean Mama Home store online). I also use an extendable duster for cobwebs and hard-to-reach ceilings and corners. Switch to a natural beeswax cream to polish and condition wood furniture monthly or as needed.

Looking for the best way to dust? Work from the top down, and quickly go through the house, dusting all the hard surfaces, any staircases and railings, the TVs, and the furniture. Do what you can within fifteen minutes. If you have extra time (beyond that fifteen minutes), add a deep-clean dusting with polish or fit in rotating cleaning tasks that don't need to be accomplished every week, like dusting light fixtures or ceiling fans.

Wednesday: Vacuuming Day

Wednesday is the day to clean up the dust from Tuesday—simple as that. Move quickly: start on the top floor if you have a multilevel home, with the room that's the farthest away from the stairs. If you have a one-level home, start at the corner farthest from the front door. Vacuum bedrooms, bathrooms, hallways, stairs, and then the lowest level. The main goal of vacuuming is to get the dust and dirt out of your home by doing a thorough job once a week. Vacuum in between as needed, but a weekly vacuuming ensures that all the dust and pet hair is picked up and the floors are ready for washing tomorrow.

Thursday: Floor Washing Day

Yes, it would be optimal to vacuum and wash floors all on the same day, but I just don't have that kind of time, and I'm guessing you don't either. So I split the tasks up. Alternatively, you can do one floor or section of your house on Wednesday and the other on Thursday. The point is to make sure that your floors are clean by the end of the day on Thursday.

There are so many floor-cleaning products and tools on the market—find one that fits your budget and you'll enjoy using. I recommend floor tools that have removable microfiber mop heads or pads. If you like making your own cleaners or want to choose what goes in your floor cleaner, choose a refillable spray mop. If you use a washable microfiber mop head or pad, dampen it first with warm water. The water will help it glide over your floors, making it easier to use, and it will more quickly clean your floors.

What's the best way to wash hard-surface floors? Start at the farthest corner in the room and wash left to right until you wash yourself out of the room. Rinse your mop head or microfiber pad frequently to avoid streaking and dullness. Working quickly and efficiently, you'll be able to get this often-dreaded task done weekly. If you find that washing the floors weekly is a little hard for you to keep up with, you can tackle one section of the house one week and another section of the house the next week. For instance, bathrooms one week and the kitchen the next week, or the first floor one week and second floor the next. Don't be afraid to experiment to see what works with your schedule and cleaning style.

Friday: Catchall Day

Think of Friday as a day to get caught up with any other homekeeping tasks and to start the weekend with a clean house. Depending on the day and week, I use Fridays to plan menus, pay bills, do laundry, complete rotating cleaning tasks, and if I'm caught up, I reward myself by taking the day off. You'll find that the weekend is so much more enjoyable if you're truly relaxed and not thinking about any nagging chores and cleaning that you "should" be doing.

Saturday: Sheets and Towels Day

On this day, wash a load or two of towels and one or two loads of sheets. I find that if I start right away in the morning, by early afternoon I have clean sheets on the beds and clean towels folded and put away. It isn't a nonstop Saturday of laundry. I just tend to the laundry when it needs to be switched from the washer to the dryer and then from the dryer to folded and put away.

Sunday: Just the Daily Tasks

Sunday is a day of rest at our house, and I love that there aren't any cleaning tasks to complete. I do daily tasks—make beds, check floors, wipe counters, declutter, and I do one load of laundry and a little planning for the upcoming week—but that's it. Relax and enjoy your Sunday. You'll feel refreshed and ready for the week ahead.

Acknowledgments

This book is what I wish I had read twenty years ago. I hope you're reading it at just the right time in your life!

For my family, thank you for your love and support and for putting up with all that comes with being an author.

For you, the reader, they say it's the little things that are really the big things after all, and I couldn't agree more. Little steps, small changes, have added up to a big impact over time in our home. I hope you give yourself grace and time to put these little but oh-so-big changes into place in your home.

A big thank you to my agent, Maria Ribas, for all your support. It's been amazing writing three books with you by my side!

For Katy Hamilton and the rest of the team at HarperOne, thank you for all your guidance and support. You've made this process so enjoyable!

To Bliss and Tell Branding Company, thank you for providing the design and vision for Clean Mama.

Above all, I am so thankful for God's provision turning my little dream into something greater than I could have ever imagined.

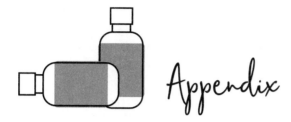

Brands and Products to Trust

I've brand-dropped throughout the book, but this is your go-to section for safe products and brands that I've vetted. These are my favorites! Please note that at the time of print, I've checked that these products are safe, but as I've pointed out, companies and standards change, so please check for yourself if you have any questions regarding safety. Hopefully you now know where to go to do your own research and are equipped to purchase the best products for your home and family, but I know it's so much easier when you have solid recommendations to start with.

Of course, there are plenty of ways to make common household products for your home, and I've given you dozens of recipes and methods for how to do so throughout the pages of this book. I've also created a page on my website for you to consult when you're putting together your safe home products. I'll update it with new products as they become available and with the latest findings. Go here to check out the safe shop: CleanMama.net/healthy-home-products.

Cleaning

Here are some places to find cleaning supplies, ingredients, and tools to make cleaning your home effective and safe.

CLEAN MAMA HOME—I have a small online shop filled with my favorite natural tools and cleaning products, with everything from glass spray bottles to wool dryer balls. (cleanmamahome.net)

AMAZON—You probably already know that you can find pretty much everything on Amazon. It's a great place to search for products that you might not find locally, and with Prime shipping, you can pretty much have anything in a day or two. (amazon.com)

AUNT FANNIE'S—If you like cleaning with vinegar, Aunt Fannie's sells scented versions for you. (auntfannies.com)

BETTER LIFE—This company is routinely at the top of the list for safe products to use all across the home. I recommend their cleaning wipes, liquid detergent, furniture spray, dish soap, and general spray cleaners. (cleanhappens.com)

BULK APOTHECARY—I use this supplier for raw materials to make specialty items like soaps, scrubs, and other home goods. They sell everything from beeswax to muslin bags and essential oils. (bulkapothecary.com)

DR. BRONNER'S—The brand that made castile soap famous. I also recommend Sal Suds cleaning concentrate from Dr. Bronner's. (drbronner.com)

EO AND EVERYONE—My favorite brands for hand soap. They don't use any artificial fragrance (just essential oils), are plant based, and don't include parabens. (eoproducts.com)

ESSENTIAL OILS—Plant Therapy, doTERRA, and Young Living are brands that I use and recommend. If you're looking to use essential oils for cleaning and diffusing, as I talk about throughout the book, make sure they are *pure* essential oils and that you're purchasing from a reliable source. (planttherapy.com, doterra.com, and youngliving.com)

FULL CIRCLE HOME—This company has quite a few eco-smart solutions for the kitchen and bath, like scrub brushes and cleaning tools, but they also carry products for composting as well as reusable storage and shopping bags. (fullcirclehome.com)

MIELE—This is my favorite brand for vacuum cleaners with bags and HEPA filters. They are fabulous at getting and keeping the dirt contained. (mieleusa.com)

MOLLY'S SUDS—They make my favorite laundry soap and oxygen whitener. These are safe and third-party tested to be just as effective as conventional brands. Molly's Suds makes some products for Clean Mama Home—that's how much I love and trust them! (mollyssuds.com)

ODE TO CLEAN—Effective cleaning wipes made entirely from plants and using Bioperoxide—love these for when you need a cleaning wipe! (odetoclean.com)

REBEL GREEN—I love Rebel Green's veggie wash and window cleaner, and they have fabulous bamboo toilet paper and paper towels that rival other brands. (rebelgreen.com)

THRIVE MARKET—I place an order with Thrive no less than monthly and love their homekeeping product selection as well as their food and pantry options. You can find quite a few of the products I mention in this book on the Thrive Market site. (thrivemarket.com)

TOOLS—I love old-fashioned wood-handled scrub brushes, brooms, and home tools. Redecker and Iris Hantverk are my favorite brands for natural tools. Look for these beautifully crafted brushes online, at your favorite utilitarian home store, or on Amazon. (redecker.de/en and irishantverk.se/en)

WHOLE FOODS—I love shopping at Whole Foods and find some products I wouldn't have found other places. I appreciate that they rate the products in their store using their own Eco-Scale—the idea is that you can choose how "green" you want to clean.[1] They rate their products in colors: green (safest), yellow, orange, and finally red (not carried). This is super helpful when you're at the store trying to decide what's safe and what's not. (wholefoodsmarket.com)

Cleaning Concentrates

If you want one cleaner for everything in your home, here are a few that pretty much fit the bill. Safe and effective, these concentrates just require a couple of spray bottles and a scrub brush. Some can be used as laundry and dish soap as well.

BRANCH BASICS CONCENTRATE—unscented (branchbasics.com)

EO ALL-PURPOSE SOAP—lemon scent (eoproducts.com)

DR. BRONNER'S SAL SUDS—light pine scent (drbronner.com)

YOUNG LIVING THIEVES HOUSEHOLD CLEANER CONCENTRATE—lemon and spice scent (youngliving.com)

Personal Care

If you're looking to invest in some better beauty and personal care products, check out this list of companies with safe products to make you look and feel good!

ACURE—A wide selection of high-quality makeup, lotions, and baby products. (acure.com)

ALAFFIA—Facial soaps, moisturizers, body wash, serums, and other products for the whole family. (alaffia.com)

BEAUTYCOUNTER—As I mentioned in chapter 10, if you want a quick and easy way to swap out your toiletries and makeup products, this brand is it. I love their lip glosses, makeup, kid products, hair care products, and sunscreens. (beautycounter.com)

BUMBLE & BEE ORGANIC—Organic lotions, deodorants, lip balms, and shower gels. (bumbleandbee.com)

DIFFUSERS—Any essential oil online shop will carry diffusers. They can be pricey. Check the size of room you can fill with the diffuser and check the duration of the diffusing. I like six or more hours of diffusing and a larger room option. Plant Therapy, doTERRA, and Young Living all have a variety of diffusers that I have tested and recommend. You also can find diffusers on the internet—my favorite brand is VicTsing. (planttherapy.com, doterra.com, and youngliving.com)

DR. BRONNER'S—Along with their cleaning supplies, they sell soaps, lotions, and toothpastes. (drbronner.com)

EO AND EVERYONE—In addition to hand soap, these two related brands also have a three-in-one body wash/shampoo/bubble bath product in a few different naturally derived scents, as well as body lotions and salt soaks. (eoproducts.com)

HELLO—Natural and effective oral care products, such as toothpaste—a safe choice for the whole family. (hello-products.com)

THE HONEST COMPANY—Safe beauty and baby products, especially well known for their diapers and wipes. (honest.com)

LOLA—Feminine care products made with organic materials. (mylola.com)

MOUNTAIN ROSE HERBS—A wonderful source for personal and body care products, essential oils, and DIY ingredients, tools, and containers. (mountainroseherbs.com)

NATIVE—Aluminum-free, paraben-free deodorants made in the USA. (nativecos.com)

PRIMALLY PURE—Nontoxic skin care and deodorants. (primallypure.com)

ROCKY MOUNTAIN SOAP COMPANY—This Canadian company is 100 percent natural and toxin-free. They carry bar soaps, body washes, baby products, sunscreens, and more. (rockymountainsoap.com)

SCHMIDT'S—My favorite choice for toothpaste and deodorant. (schmidtsnaturals.com)

SHEA MOISTURE—Lotions, shampoos, and body washes made with all natural ingredients. (sheamoisture.com)

TUBBY TODD BATH COMPANY—A selection of natural bath products, such as lotions and soaps, for the kids. (tubbytodd .com)

Kitchen

I mentioned a lot of changes and swaps that can be made in the kitchen. Here are some places to start:

BALL CANNING JARS—Use these jars for pantry and dry storage. (ball.com)

BEE'S WRAP—Makers of a natural, reusable, and compostable alternative to plastic wrap, made from GOTS-certified organic cotton, sustainably sourced beeswax, organic jojoba oil, and tree resin. (beeswrap.com)

IF YOU CARE—This company makes ecofriendly parchment paper, waxed paper, foil, bags, and more. Their paper products are chlorine-free, their foil is 100 percent recycled aluminum, and they now carry nonstick parchment roasting bags that are free of petroleum-based plastic. (ifyoucare.com)

LE CREUSET—Beautiful enameled cast-iron cookware and bakeware that will last you a lifetime (and most products even come with a limited lifetime warranty). (lecreuset.com)

LIBBEY—An easy to find option for glassware and storage, Libbey has been around for years. (libbey.com)

LODGE—Made in the United States, these cast-iron pans are well made, come preseasoned, and will last generations. (lodgemfg.com)

LUNCHSKINS—I love these recyclable and resealable paper bags for kids' lunches and food on the go. They also have reusable Velcro and zipper-top varieties. The darling prints on the bags make them even more fun to use. (lunchskins.com)

PYREX—Don't you just love Pyrex? This nearly impossible to break glassware is an all-purpose solution for many things in the kitchen, and they have some wonderful reusable storage options. (pyrexware.com)

STASHER BAGS—I love these silicone bags in lieu of plastic sandwich bags (I use these for storage, not heating). They come in lots of fun colors and a few different sizes, perfect for food storage needs. (stasherbag.com)

Electronics

SAFESLEEVE—My favorite brand for EMF-blocking technology. I have the case for my iPhone. Their cases are cute and functional. (safesleevecases.com)

DEFENDERSHIELD—EMF- and heat-blocking laptop pad—I have this for my laptop and find that it's lightweight and easy to use. (defendershield.com)

FELIX GRAY—Blue-light-blocking glasses—these eliminate eyestrain from devices. I use them when I'm on my computer for extended periods of time. (shopfelixgray.com)

TECH WELLNESS—An online company that promotes unplugging daily from technology. They also have excellent resources for the safe use of technology and for blocking EMFs. (techwellness.com)

Resources for More Information

EWG.ORG—Environmental Working Group is an organization that offers information on food and household product safety.

EWG.ORG/SKINDEEP—This is EWG's database for cosmetics.

EWG'S HEALTHY LIVING APP—This app allows you to scan products on the go for their safety.

GREEN BUILDING SUPPLY—If you're looking to build or replace flooring in your home, this company, out of Iowa, is an amazing resource, and they ship nationwide. Look into safe alternatives before choosing any brand. (greenbuildingsupply.com)

MADESAFE.ORG—This organization evaluates and certifies household products.

THINK DIRTY APP—This is another app that will allow you to scan products on the go for their safety.

The small changes you make will result in a big impact in your home and in your neighborhood too. I hope you find solutions to help you create the oasis you have always dreamed of walking into. May your home be safe, clean, and a haven for you and your family.

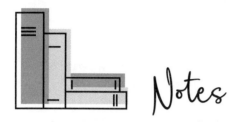

Notes

CHAPTER 1: IS YOUR HOME MAKING YOU SICK?

1. According to *Chemistry World*, in the forty years since TSCA was formed, just over 200 out of 85,000-plus chemicals have actually been tested and assessed. Further, only 5 classes of chemicals have been banned—these include asbestos, hexavalent chromium in A/C units, and halogenated solvents in aerosols. Rebecca Trager, "Explainer: Toxic Substances Control Act," *Chemistry World*, June 10, 2016, https://www.chemistryworld .com/news/explainer-toxic-substances-control-act/1010187.article; Environmental Protection Agency, "EPA Marks Chemical Safety Milestone on 1st Anniversary of Lautenberg Chemical Safety Act," June 22, 2017, https://www.epa.gov/newsreleases /epa-marks-chemical-safety-milestone-1st-anniversary-lautenberg-chemical-safety-act.

2. Natural Resources Defense Council, "Toxic Chemicals," https://www.nrdc.org/issues /toxic-chemicals.

3. Ian Urbina, "Think Those Chemicals Have Been Tested?" *New York Times*, April 13, 2013, https://www.nytimes.com/2013/04/14/sunday-review/think-those-chemicals-have-been -tested.html.

4. Made Safe, "About Us," https://madesafe.org/about/about-us/.

5. Environmental Protection Agency, "The Inside Story: A Guide to Indoor Air Quality," https://www.epa.gov/indoor-air-quality-iaq/inside-story-guide-indoor-air-quality.

6. American Thoracic Society, "Women Who Clean at Home or Work Face Increased Lung Function Decline, Study Finds," ScienceDaily, February 16, 2018, https://www.sciencedaily .com/releases/2018/02/180216084912.htm.

7. President's Cancer Panel, "Reducing Environmental Cancer Risk: What We Can Do Now," annual report 2008–2009, https://deainfo.nci.nih.gov/advisory/pcp/annualReports/pcp08 -09rpt/PCP_Report_08-09_508.pdf.

8. Environmental Working Group, "Body Burden: The Pollution in Newborns," July 14, 2005, https://www.ewg.org/research/body-burden-pollution-newborns#.Wr4Rl7aZM62.

CHAPTER 2: WHAT IS IN YOUR CLEANING SUPPLIES?

1. National Science Foundation, "Organic Labeling Requirements," http://www.nsf.org /consumer-resources/cooking-cleaning-food-safety/organic/organic-labeling -requirements.

2. "Organic Labeling Requirements," http://www.nsf.org/consumer-resources/cooking -cleaning-food-safety/organic/organic-labeling-requirements.

3. Greener Choices, "'Natural' Not Meaningful," *Consumer Reports*, last modified September 6, 2017, http://greenerchoices.org/2016/11/16/natural-label-review/.

4. Cruelty Free International, *The Leaping Bunny Certification: FAQs,* http://www.oneplanet network.org/sites/default/files/introduction_to_leaping_bunny_faqs_2017.pdf.

5. Leaping Bunny Program, "The Leaping Bunny Logo," http://www.leapingbunny.org /content/leaping-bunny-logo.

6. Non GMO Project, "Product Verification," https://www.nongmoproject.org/product-verification/.

7. Non GMO Project, "GMO Facts," https://www.nongmoproject.org/gmo-facts/.

8. Certified B Corporation, "Certification," https://www.bcorporation.net/become-a-b-corp /how-to-become-a-b-corp.

9. Melaleuca the Wellness Company, "What's in Your Home Products?," *Healthy Cells Magazine*, March 4, 2014, http://www.healthycellsmagazine.com/articles/what-s-in -your-home-products.

10. Environmental Working Group, "Statement of Jane Houlihan on Cosmetics Safety," July 25, 2008, https://www.ewg.org/news/testimony-official-correspondence/statement -jane-houlihan-cosmetics-safety#.W1TtJi_MyDc.

11. ChemicalSafetyFacts.org, "Ammonia," https://www.chemicalsafetyfacts.org/ammonia/.

12. Environmental Working Group, "Ammonium Hydroxide," https://www.ewg.org/guides /substances/338#.WzDpdS-ZOWY.

13. Alison Kodjak, "FDA Bans 19 Chemicals Used in Antibacterial Soaps," Your Health, National Public Radio, September 2, 2106, https://www.npr.org/sections/health -shots/2016/09/02/492394717/fda-bans-19-chemicals-used-in-antibacterial-soaps.

14. Centers for Disease Control and Prevention, "Facts About Benzene," https://emergency .cdc.gov/agent/benzene/basics/facts.asp.

15. Dr. Axe, "Dangers of Bleach + NEVER Mix Bleach with These 3 Cleaning Ingredients," https://draxe.com/dangers-of-bleach/.

16. Environmental Protection Agency, *Technical Fact Sheet—1,4-Dioxane*, November 2017, https://www.epa.gov/sites/production/files/2014-03/documents/ffrro_factsheet _contaminant_14-dioxane_january2014_final.pdf.

17. Environmental Working Group, "1-4-Dioxane," EWG's Skin Deep, https://www.ewg.org /skindeep/ingredient/726331/1%2C4-DIOXANE/#.

18. Environmental Protection Agency, *Health and Environmental Effects Profile for Formaldehyde*, EPA/600/x-85/362, Environmental Criteria and Assessment Office, 1988; American Cancer Society, "What Causes Cancer? Formaldehyde," May 23, 2014, https://www.cancer.org/cancer/cancer-causes/formaldehyde.html.

19. *Encyclopedia Britannica*, s.v. "Urea-Formaldehyde Resin," https://www.britannica.com /science/urea-formaldehyde-resin.

20. Steve Vogel, "New TSA Uniforms Trigger a Rash of Complaints," *Washington Post*, January 5, 2009, http://www.washingtonpost.com/wp-dyn/content/article/2009/01/05 /AR2009010502146.html?noredirect=on.

21. J. D. Thrasher, A. Broughton, and R. Madison, "Immune Activation and Autoantibodies in Humans with Long-Term Inhalation Exposure to Formaldehyde," *Archive of Environmental Health* 45, no. 4 (1990): 217–23.

22. Dr. Mercola, "10 Sources for Endocrine Disrupters and How to Avoid Them," Mercola. com, July 15, 2015, https://articles.mercola.com/sites/articles/archive/2015/07/15/10 -common-sources-endocrine-disruptors.aspx.

23. R. Scheer and D. Moss, "Should People Be Concerned About Parabens in Beauty Products?" EarthTalk, *Scientific American*, https://www.scientificamerican.com/article /should-people-be-concerned-about-parabens-in-beauty-products/.

24. National Center for Biotechnology Information, PubChem Open Chemistry Database, "Phenol," https://pubchem.ncbi.nlm.nih.gov/compound/phenol#section=Top.

25. Agency for Toxic Substances and Disease Registry, "Toxic Substances Portal—Phenol," https://www.atsdr.cdc.gov/mmg/mmg.asp?id=144&tid=27.

26. O. Andrukhova, S. Slavic, A. Smorodchenko, U. Zeitz, V. Shalhoub, B. Lanske, E. E. Pohl, and R. G. Erben, "FGF23 Regulates Renal Sodium Handling and Blood Pressure," *EMBO Molecular Medicine* (2014): e201303716, http://embomolmed.embopress.org/content/early/2014/05/05/emmm.201303716.

27. Campaign for Safe Cosmetics, "Phthalates," http://www.safecosmetics.org/get-the-facts/chemicals-of-concern/phthalates/.

28. Environmental Working Group, EWG's Skin Deep Cosmetics Database, "Sodium Lauryl Sulfate," https://www.ewg.org/skindeep/ingredient/706110/SODIUM_LAURYL_SULFATE/#.W1UtUC_MyDc.

29. Invisible Disabilities Association, "Why Go Fragrance Free?" https://invisibledisabilities.org/ida-books-pamphlets/chemicalsensitivities/whygofragrancefree/; Roddy Scheer and Doug Moss, "Scent of Danger: Are There Toxic Ingredients in Perfumes and Colognes?," EarthTalk, *Scientific American*, https://www.scientificamerican.com/article/toxic-perfumes-and-colognes/.

30. Federal Trade Commission, "Fair Packaging and Labeling Act," https://www.ftc.gov/enforcement/rules/rulemaking-regulatory-reform-proceedings/fair-packaging-labeling-act.

31. Campaign for Safe Cosmetics, "Fragrance," http://www.safecosmetics.org/get-the-facts/chemicals-of-concern/fragrance/.

32. Environmental Protection Agency, "Xylenes," updated January 2000, https://www.epa.gov/sites/production/files/2016-09/documents/xylenes.pdf.

33. Agency for Toxic Substance and Disease Registry, Division of Toxicology and Environmental Medicine, *Public Health Statement: Xylene,* August 2007, https://www.atsdr.cdc.gov/ToxProfiles/tp71-c1-b.pdf.

CHAPTER 3: THE TOXIC TEN AND WHOLE HOME SWAPS

1. Environmental Working Group, "Shopper's Guide to the Pesticides in Produce," https://www.ewg.org/foodnews/.

2. Daniel Simmons, "Organic Lawn Care Products Require Patience," Angie's List, https://www.angieslist.com/articles/organic-lawn-care-products-require-patience.htm.

3. Environmental Working Group, "EWG's Guide to Bug Repellants: Protecting from Zika

Virus," July 17, 2018, https://www.ewg.org/research/ewgs-guide-bug-repellents-age -zika/what-you-can-do-about-zika#.WymrAy-ZPOQ.

4. University of Washington, "Scented Laundry Products Emit Hazardous Chemicals Through Dryer Vents," ScienceDaily, August 24, 2011, https://www.sciencedaily.com /releases/2011/08/110824091537.htm.

5. Dr. Axe, "Stop Using Dryer Sheets Immediately!" https://draxe.com/dryer-sheets/.

6. Food and Drug Administration, "Consumer Updates," https://www.fda.gov/For Consumers/ConsumerUpdates/default.htm.

7. Bruce Fellman, "The Problem with Plastics," *Environment: Yale* (Fall 2009), http:// environment.yale.edu/magazine/fall2009/the-problem-with-plastics/.

8. Bee's Wrap, "About Us," https://www.beeswrap.com/pages/about-us.

9. USPIRG, "FDA's BPA Ban: A Small, Late Step In the Right Direction," blog, July 17, 2013, https://uspirg.org/blogs/blog/usp/fda's-bpa-ban-small-late-step-right-direction.

10. R. Scheer and D. Moss, "Avoid Harsh Chemicals in Commercial Air Fresheners with Homemade Alternatives," EarthTalk, *Scientific American,* https://www.scientific american.com/article/nontoxic-air-fresheners/.

CHAPTER 4: THE SECRET TO GOING ORGANIC WITHOUT SPENDING A FORTUNE

1. Heidi Nickerson, "How Much Money Does an Average Family Spend on Cleaning Products in a Year?," The Nest, accessed September 6, 2018, https://budgeting.thenest .com/much-money-average-family-spend-cleaning-products-year-23539.html.

CHAPTER 5: THE WHOLE HOME DETOX PANTRY

1. Plant Therapy, "KidSafe," https://www.planttherapy.com/kid-safe.

2. ASPCA News, "Is the Latest Home Trend Harmful to Your Pets? What You Need to Know!," January 17, 2018, https://www.aspca.org/news/latest-home-trend-harmful-your -pets-what-you-need-know.

CHAPTER 7: FIVE-MINUTE HIGH-IMPACT CHANGES

1. Cleaning Industry Research Institute, "Study Reveals High Bacteria Levels on Footwear," last modified May 3, 2008, https://www.ciriscience.org/a_96-Study-Reveals-High -Bacteria-Levels-on-Footwear.

2. Greg Seaman, "The Top 10 Plants for Removing Indoor Toxins," Eartheasy, September 6,

2017, http://learn.eartheasy.com/2009/05/the-top-10-plants-for-removing-indoor
-toxins/.

3. NASA Spinoff. "Plants Clean Air and Water for Indoor Environments," https://spinoff
.nasa.gov/Spinoff2007/ps_3.html.

4. Environmental Protection Agency, "The Inside Story: A Guide to Indoor Air Quality,"
https://www.epa.gov/indoor-air-quality-iaq/inside-story-guide-indoor-air-quality.

CHAPTER 9: KITCHEN

1. Roni Caryn Rabin, "Chemicals in Food May Harm Children, Pediatricians' Group Says,"
New York Times, July 23, 2018, https://www.nytimes.com/2018/07/23/well/chemicals
-food-children-health.html.

2. Vanessa Vadim, "What's the Safest Cookware?" Mother Nature Network, September 23,
2015, https://www.mnn.com/food/healthy-eating/questions/whats-the-safest-cookware;
American Cancer Society, "What Causes Cancer? Teflon and Perfluorooctanoic Acid
(PFOA)," January 5, 2016, https://www.cancer.org/cancer/cancer-causes/teflon-and
-perfluorooctanoic-acid-pfoa.html.

3. Dr. Edward Group, "Are Microwaves Dangerous to Your Health?" Global Healing Center,
March 22, 2017, https://www.globalhealingcenter.com/natural-health/are-microwaves
-dangerous-to-your-health/.

4. On the effects of what we eat and how it's traced to diseases, see the book *In Defense
of Food: An Eater's Manifesto,* by Michael Pollan, (New York: Penguin, 2009).

CHAPTER 10: BATHROOM

1. Ian Urbina, "Think Those Chemicals Have Been Tested?" *New York Times,* April 13, 2013,
https://www.nytimes.com/2013/04/14/sunday-review/think-those-chemicals-have-been
-tested.html.

2. Sephora, "Clean at Sephora," https://www.sephora.com/clean-beauty-products.

3. Food and Drug Administration, "FDA Authority Over Cosmetics: How Cosmetics
Are Not FDA-Approved, but Are FDA-Regulated," https://www.fda.gov/Cosmetics
/GuidanceRegulation/LawsRegulations/ucm074162.htm.

4. Beautycounter, "Our Story," https://www.beautycounter.com/our-story.

5. Beautycounter, "Our Story."

6. Dr. Edward Group, "The Dangers of Fluoride," Global Healing Center, November 16, 2015, https://www.globalhealingcenter.com/natural-health/how-safe-is-fluoride/.

7. Organic Facts, "16 Proven Health Benefits & Uses of Coconut Oil," https://www.organicfacts.net/health-benefits/oils/health-benefits-of-coconut-oil.html.

8. Environmental Protection Agency, "Volatilization Rates from Water to Indoor Air Phase II," https://cfpub.epa.gov/ncea/risk/recordisplay.cfm?deid=20677.

9. Underground Health Reporter, "Dangers of Chlorine in Your Shower," http://undergroundhealthreporter.com/dangers-of-chlorine-in-your-shower; Lawrence K. Altman, "Tiny Cancer Risk in Chlorinated Water," *New York Times*, July 1, 1992, https://www.nytimes.com/1992/07/01/us/tiny-cancer-risk-in-chlorinated-water.html.

CHAPTER 11: LIVING AREAS

1. Markham Heid, "You Asked: Can My Couch Give Me Cancer?" Time.com, August 24, 2016, http://time.com/4462892/couch-cancer-flame-retardants/.

CHAPTER 12: BEDROOMS

1. Joe Palca, "The Dirt on Dust," Morning Edition, National Public Radio, November 16, 2009, https://www.npr.org/templates/story/story.php?storyId=120252957.

2. Dr. Mercola, "What's Hiding in Your Mattress?" Mercola.com, December 30, 2015, https://articles.mercola.com/sites/articles/archive/2015/12/30/mattress-toxic-chemicals.aspx.

3. National Cancer Institute, "Cell Phones and Cancer Risk," https://www.cancer.gov/about-cancer/causes-prevention/risk/radiation/cell-phones-fact-sheet.

CHAPTER 13: LAUNDRY

1. Environmental Working Group, "Sulfuric Acid," https://www.ewg.org/guides/substances/14662-SULFURICACID#.W1X0ei_MyDc.

APPENDIX

1. Whole Foods, "Eco-Scale: Giving New Meaning to Cleaning," https://www.wholefoodsmarket.com/eco-scale-our-commitment.

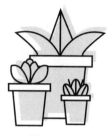

Index